TEACHING YOGA WITH VERBAL CUES

PRIMARY SERIES

David Garrigues

Editor, Joy Marzec
Designer/Contributor, Joanna Darlington

Copyright

Please email asanakitchen@gmail.com if you'd like to use any of this material in a training.

All rights reserved.

No part of this publication may be reproduced, stored in a retrieval system, stored in a database and/or published in any form or by any means, electronic, mechanical, photocopying, recording or otherwise, without the prior written permission of the publisher.

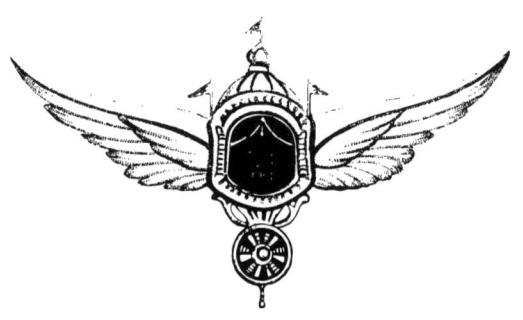

Introduction

An overwhelming fear of public speaking almost stopped me from becoming a yoga teacher. At one point, I attended several teacher trainings and I could never bring myself to volunteer, stand in front of the group, and deliver a few instructions.

I was close to despair. And then, on a whim, I decided to make a set of āsana flashcards. I got index cards, wrote the posture name on one side and the basic verbal commands for doing the pose on the other side. I quizzed myself and spoke the commands out loud as though delivering instructions to students in a class. And this odd little device gave me surprisingly effective results. I grew confident in my knowledge of yoga and eventually summoned courage to share with others.

These verbal cues are a lot like the original ones I created but also represent a crystallization of nearly 30 years of passionate teaching. I hope you find them easy to use, technically precise, and poetically inspiring! May you learn to articulate the verbal cues, use them to teach your students how to strike the immovable spot in each pose, and know the great āsana technology that helps each yogī realize their intrinsic essence as a spiritual Seer.

Jai,
David

What are Verbal Cues?

A verbal cue is a concise command that gives a clear direction to a student. They are an essential tool for a teacher and are just as important as a physical adjustment. They help the student to find actions throughout the body so they can become skillful and autonomous in expressing a pose.

Benefits of Verbal Cues

— Better understand how to deliver verbal commands and become more effective teaching the poses of the Primary Series.

— Gain expertise in voicing biomechanical alignment principles.

— Help students clarify worthy goal(s) for doing each pose.

— Teach students to activate the whole body, get every tiniest part involved in what they are doing.

— Develop skill in troubleshooting poses and help students lessen or eliminate pain.

— Help students get more control over building strength and creating flexibility.

— Help students better understand what Bandhas are and how to activate them.

— Help students to practice the inner limbs of yoga—dhāraṇā (concentration), dhyāna (meditation), samādhi (absorption).

Advanced View of Action

"Yogaścittavṛttinirodhaḥ" is the goal of yoga and is defined as a 'cessation of thought'. The word Nirodha means to cease, to stop, to arrest, and refers to the ultimate state of mind—empty, clear, uncluttered, at rest, settled, peaceful, nonreactive, spontaneous, spacious, embracing, uniting, loving, and free.

However, before you can know Nirodha there is an important middle step called, Pravṛtti or Higher thought, that involves learning to activate the mind to consciously thwart or bypass the habitual, unskillful, thoughts that usually occupy the mind.

As a teacher, these flashcards give you examples of Pravṛtti to share with your students. Each set of verbal cues gives āsana actions that will help your students clear their minds of extraneous thoughts so they can reach a state of Nirodha. In this way the goal of action is to attain a state of No Mind and this is the yogīs secret weapon that helps them respond effectively and appropriately to any and all circumstances.

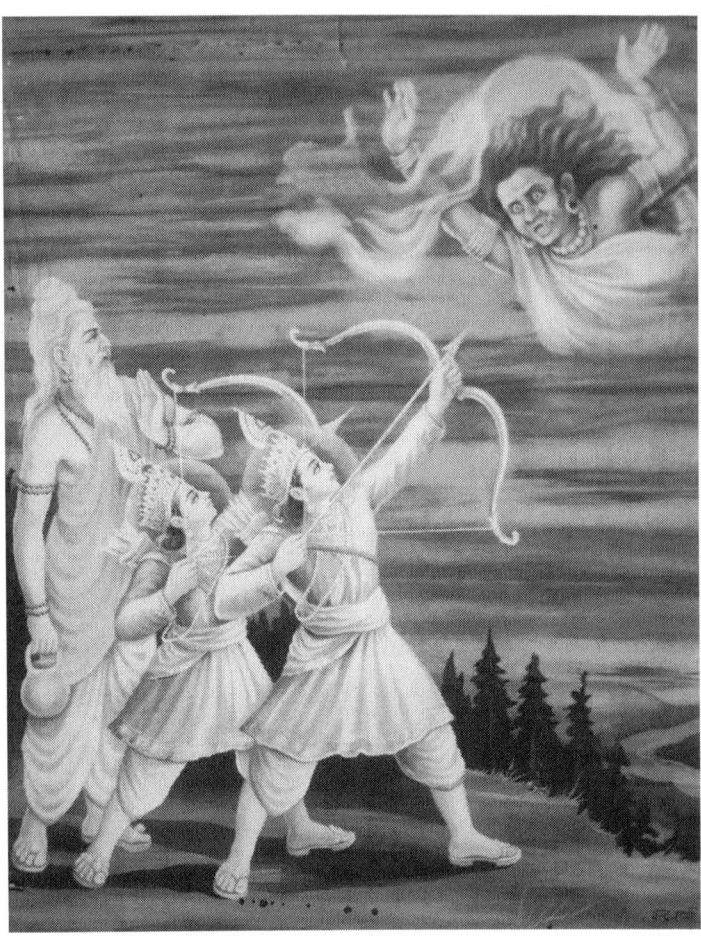

The God Rāma and his guru Vāsiṣṭha

Lord Rāma, the boy in the foreground, pulls back his bow to shoot the arrow that will kill the demon up in the sky. Rām's brother, Lakshman, and the great sage Vāsiṣṭha, stand beside him offering support.

Yoga Vasiṣṭha: Action Ślokas

— Destroy anything doubtful by the power of purity in action. If there is an increase in purified habits then there can be no fault.

— When the yogī makes a great effort and purifies her present actions, she overcomes the impurity and harm of past actions.

— Just as when two rams fight and the stronger prevails without much trouble, so there are two unequal forces of human exertion; that of the present overcomes the past.

— Whatever one strives for, that very thing is obtained through one's actions only.

— To make a perfect pot or perfect weaving (or a perfect āsana), restraint, steady calculation, and human exertion are needed.

— In this world whatever is gained is gained by self-effort; where failure is encountered it is seen that there has been slackness in the effort.

— There is no power greater than right action in the present.

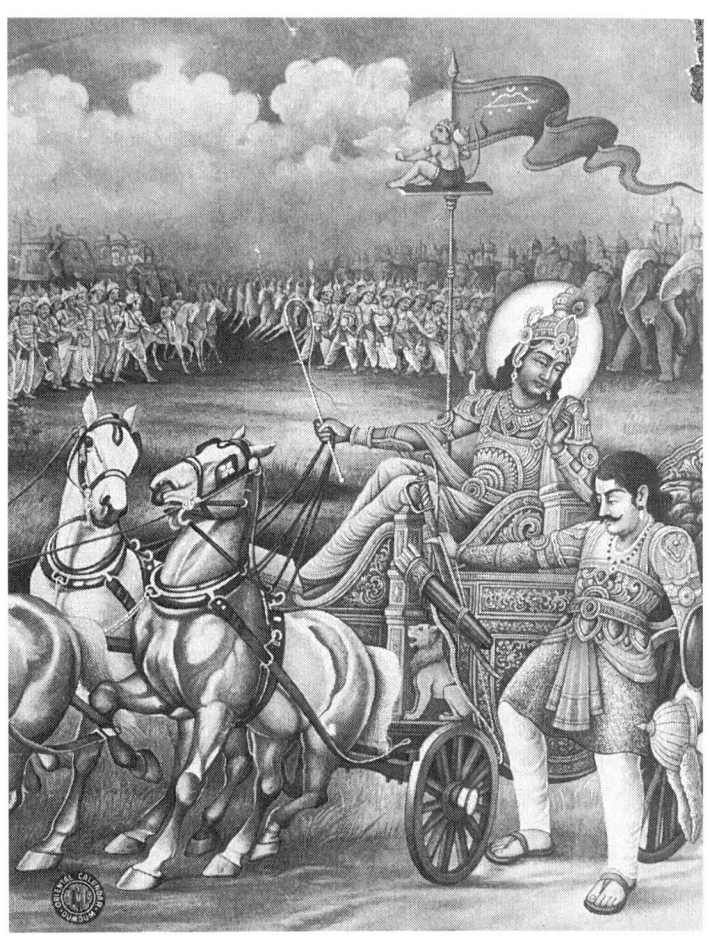

The God Kṛṣṇa and the great yogī Arjuna

This picture is set just before the start of the battle between the forces of good and evil in the epic story called the Mahābhārata. Kṛṣṇa, the chariot driver, who is also God, urges Arjuna (who symbolizes you and me) to overcome his doubt and perform actions in order to fulfill his sacred duty.

Bhagavad Gītā: Action Ślokas

— A woman cannot escape the force of action by abstaining from actions; she does not obtain success just by renunciation.
  – Ch.3, V.3

— No one exists even for an instant without performing actions; however unwilling, every being is forced to act by the qualities of nature (guṇas).
  – Ch.3, V.4

— Perform necessary action; it is more powerful than inaction; without action you even fail to sustain your own body.
  – Ch.3, V.8

— What is action? What is inaction? Even the poets are confused—what I shall teach you of action will free you from misfortune.
  – Ch.4, V.16

— One should understand action, understand wrong action, and understand inaction too; the way of action is difficult to fathom.
  – Ch.4, V.17

— The one who sees inaction in action and action in inaction is a sage.
  – Ch.4, V.18

— Having renounced attachment to action and its fruit, always happy, depending upon nothing, the yogī does nothing though always engaged in action.
  – Ch.4, V.20

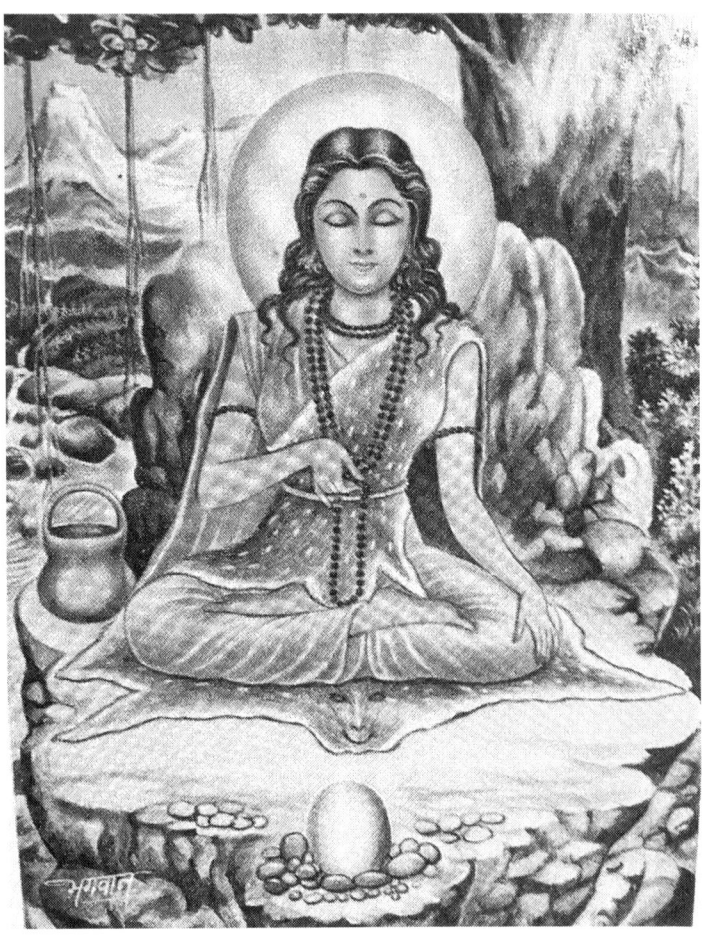

Parvati in Samadhi

The Goddess Parvati sits in Padmāsana (Full Lotus Pose) practicing Japa Mantra with prayer beads. Her outer serenity also has an intense inner dynamism. She strikes an immovable spot, stops all movements of her body and mind and yet continues to play with, rather than reject, deny, or hate the infinite pairs of opposing forces that are constantly butting up against each other within her.

Yoga Taraṅgiṇī: Action Ślokas

— Just as a falcon tied by a string can be pulled back after going away, so too the yogī draws fragmented consciousness back to unity by activating Prāṇa and Apāna Vāyus when in a pose.
  – Ch.1, V.40

— Apāna pulls on the Prāṇa and the Prāṇa pulls on the Apāna. These two forms of the Life Force are situated above and below the navel. Through skillful action the knower of yoga joins these two.
  – Ch.1, V.41

— Just as one should forcefully open a door using a key, so the yogi should penetrate the door to liberation by activating the Kuṇḍalinī.
  – Ch.1, V.51

— That place from which the great bird (Prāṇa) makes its tireless, soaring flight would verily be the Uḍḍīyāna Bandha—Belly Flying Up Lock—a lion to the elephant of death.
  – Ch.1, V.60

— The knower of yoga who drinks the ambrosia (Prāṇa, consciousness) by pressing the tongue to the roots of the teeth conquers death within half a month no doubt.
  – Ch.2, V.44

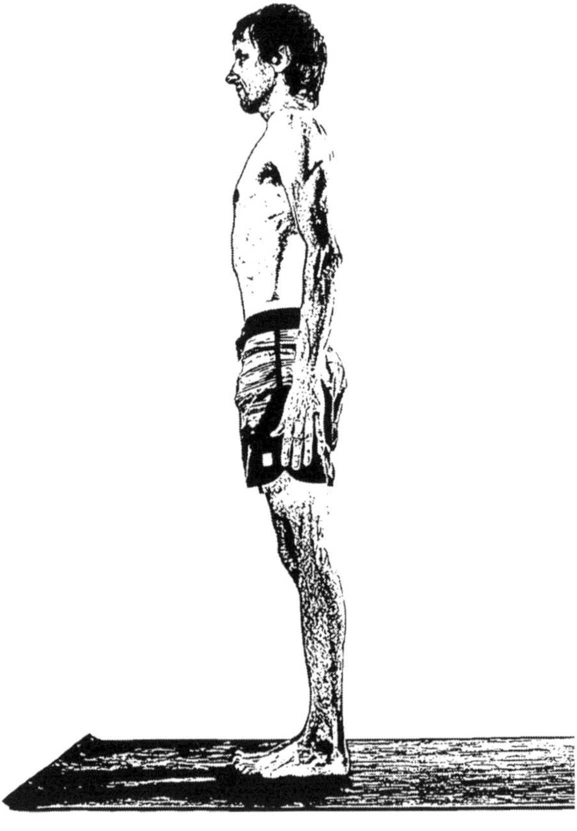

Samasthitiḥ
(Equal Standing Pose)

— Stamp the earth with your feet and ground your legs.
— Lift up your foot arches, kneecaps, quadriceps, and navel.
— Press your thighbones deeper into your legs.
— Weight your coccyx and perform Uḍḍīyāna Bandha (Belly Flying Up Gesture); tilt your pelvis to neutral.
— Broaden your chest and roll your shoulders back into the side plane.
— Lengthen the lines of your limbs by reaching down through your leg bones from hips to feet, and your arm bones from shoulders to fingers.
— Vertically align your head, torso, pelvis, legs, and feet.
— Level your chin, lift up the back of your skull, and lengthen your neck.
— Clear your palate and cast a steady gaze towards the horizon.
— Internalize your awareness; visualize your central axis as a vertical pillar of light that shines like a sun whose rays light up the entire body and the cosmos with fresh vital energy.

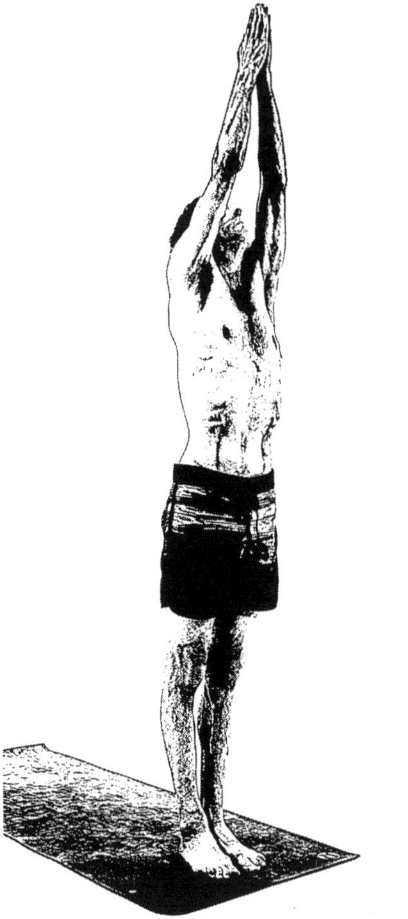

First and Ninth Positions of Sūrya Namaskāra A

(Ūrdhva Hastāsana)

— Reach vertically upward through your arms in a mighty gesture of extension; touch the sky with your fingers.

— Stamp the earth with your feet and ground your thighbones; create an immoveable lower body with roots deep in the earth.

— Vertically line up your wrists, elbows, shoulders, pelvis, knees, and ankles.

— Visualize your skeleton as a fiery column of light and charge your body with energy.

— Lift up the pit of your abdomen and expand your upper chest as you widen your back ribs and kidneys.

— Maintain length through your neck as you gaze up towards the sky past your thumbs.

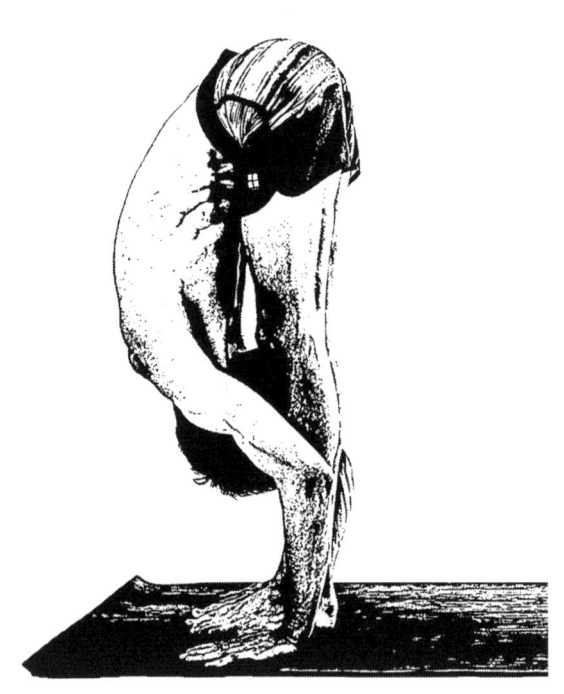

Second and Eighth Positions of Sūrya Namaskāra A
(Uttānāsana)

— Shift your body forward to the edge of imbalance.
— Stamp down through your feet and hands.
— Brace your legs and arms, fix your limbs firmly in position.
— Imagine your legs grow taller like you are standing on stilts.
— Lift up your pelvis along the vertical axis.
— Release your spine from tail to head.
— Patiently bring your torso towards your grounded legs.
— Relax your brain, clear your palate, internalize your gaze.
— Cause the steady sound of your breath to flow smoothly up and down the Glorious Middle Channel.

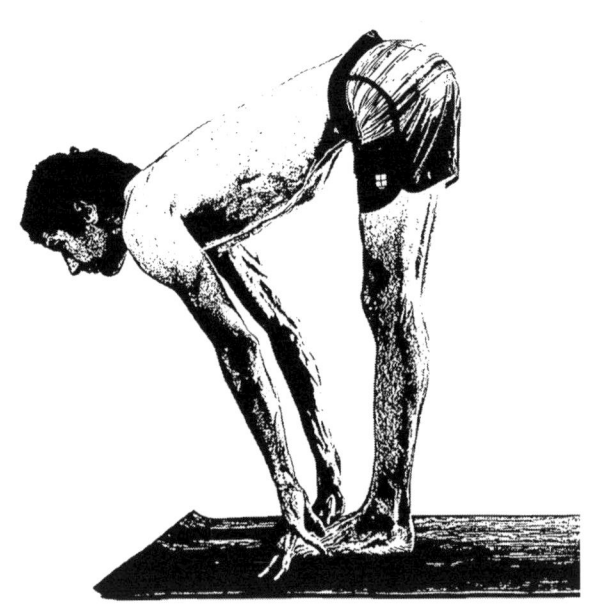

Third and Seventh Positions of Sūrya Namaskāra A
(Ardha Uttānāsana)

— Plant your feet and make your legs tall and firm.
— Lift your palms; go up on your fingertips.
— Project your spine horizontally forward and away from your fixed legs.
— Lift up your head and chest high; fully extend your arms.
— Press down and back through your fingertips.
— Lift and separate the sitting bones, press your pubic bone back.
— Set your pelvis to a neutral tilt along a horizontal axis.
— Suck your front ribs up towards the spine and lift your chest.
— Cast a confident gaze up between your eyebrows.

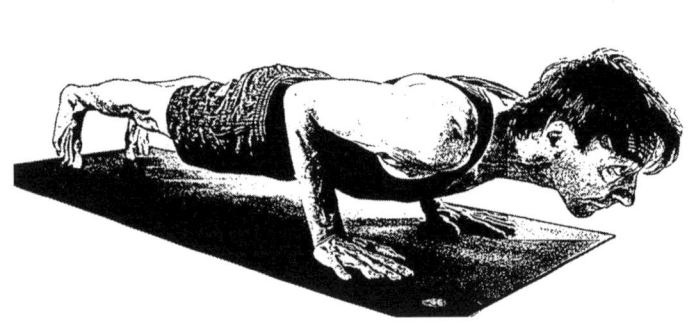

Caturaṅga Daṇḍāsana
(Four Limbed Staff Pose)

— Strike down through your hands and firmly brace your arms.

— Imagine your arms and legs are dense and compact; ready for action like loaded springs.

— Strike Samasthitiḥ; align your head, torso, pelvis, and legs into an unbreakable horizontal stick.

— Pull up your navel and strengthen your center.

— Activate the "Big 4" muscle groups that surround your center: hamstrings, quadriceps, buttocks, and abdomen.

— Widen your back ribs and suck your front ribs up towards the spine; lift the top of your sternum and widen your collarbones.

— Hover your firm body just above the earth; focus your gaze forward with steely determination.

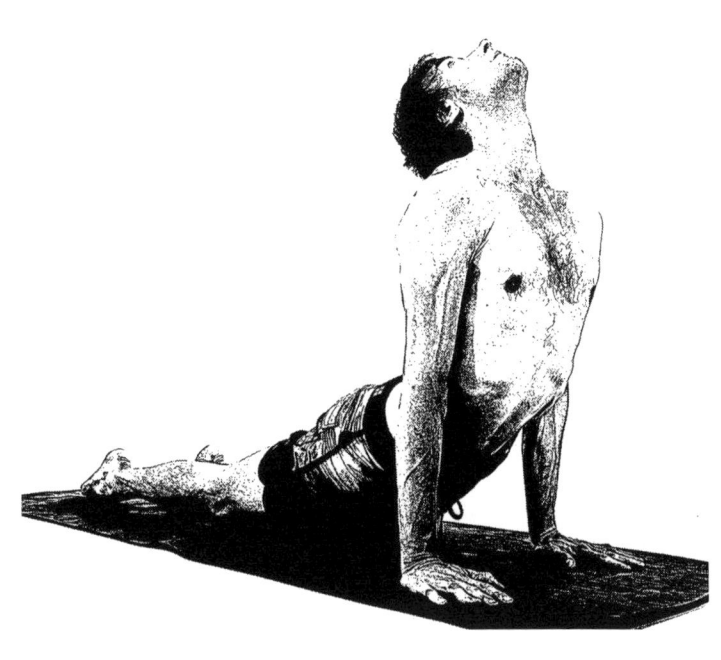

Ūrdhva Mukha Śvānāsana
(Upward Facing Dog Pose)

— Stamp down into the earth through your hands, powerfully lift up your head, and make a shapely circle with your spine.

— Reach back through your legs from hips to toes.

— Firm your buttocks and hamstrings, make your kneecaps face directly down, and fully point your toes.

— Lift your head and spine up off of your shoulder girdle, and suck your spine forward between your strong, tall arms.

— Create maximum contrast between lifting up your spine and stamping down through your arms and hands.

— Anchor your legs; use their fixed position as leverage to suck your chest forward and increase the curve of your spine.

— Think: chest forward, head and legs back.

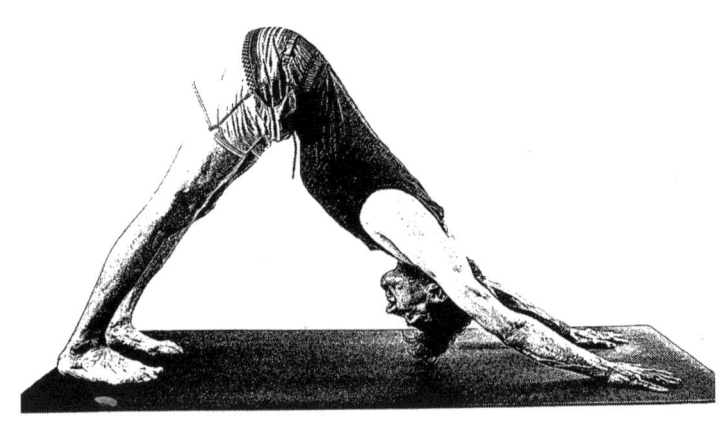

Adho Mukha Śvānāsana
(Downward Facing Dog Pose)

— Press your hands down into the earth and root back through your thighs.

— Project your pelvis up and your thighs back in opposition to pressing your hands down into the ground.

— Lift your sitting bones and press back through your pubic bone; tilt your pelvis to neutral in agreement with your spine's diagonal line.

— Align your three main body masses to create integrity along the diagonal line that spans from your pelvic floor to the crown of your head, and through your extended arms.

— Fix your legs and arms in position, suck your front ribs up into your body, and allow your spine to dip down into your torso.

— Imagine your spine is like a suspension bridge cable; allow the column to swoop down from tail to head supported by your stuborn, unmoving arms and legs.

— Maintain the strength of your limbs and allow your head and spine to come closer to the ground as you stay riveted in position.

— Cast a steady gaze towards your thighs, pelvis, or navel.

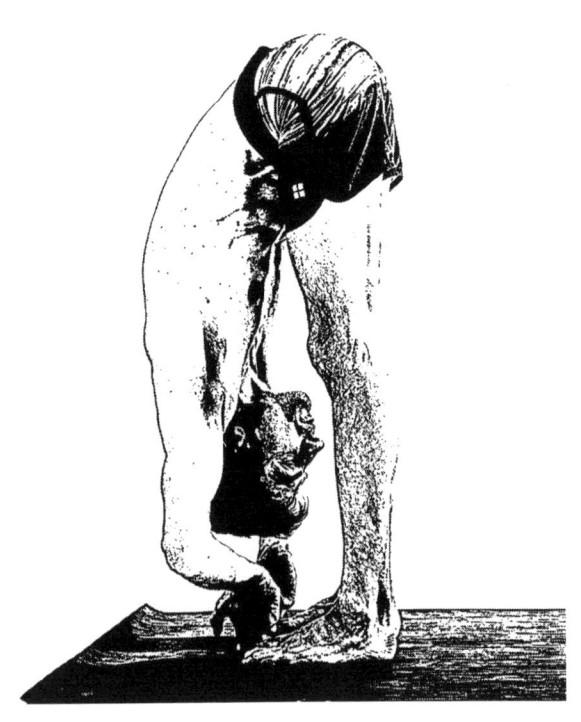

Pādāṅguṣṭhāsana
(Big Toe Pose)

— Pull up on your big toes with your fingers and stamp your fingers down with your toes.
— Lift your hips and lengthen your legs.
— Vertically align your pelvis, knees, and ankles.
— Hug the thigh muscles to the bones; press your thighbones deeper into your legs.
— Release the spine; drape the torso over your sturdy legs.
— Create your forward bend on the edge of imbalance; shift forward to a precipice and hold steady.
— Suck your belly into a hollow; catch a mudrā.
— Gradually bring your torso towards your rooted, unmoving legs; breathe freely.
— Perceive your inner world; internalize your senses; steady your mind; delight in absorption.
— Be happy upside down; explore the world inside your body; create a playful, inverted meditation seat.
— Circulate Prāṇa through your body in a loop; start at your feet, go up your legs to your pelvis, and down your torso through your arms to your hands.

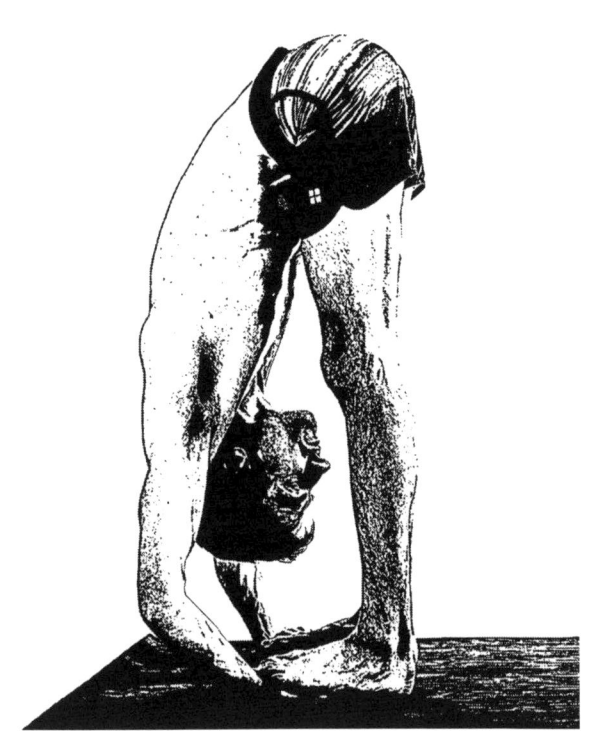

Pāda Hastāsana
(Hand to Foot Pose)

— Press your feet down onto your hands with confidence.

— Fearlessly take to this upside down jack knife shape.

— Pull up through your arms and lift up your pelvis.

— Lengthen your legs and elongate your spine.

— Gently will your torso to move closer to your stubborn, fixed legs.

— Shift forward to the edge of imbalance; find the immovable spot in a play of dynamic forces.

— Suck your belly into a hollow; strike Uḍḍīyāna Bandha.

— Listen to your breath; make an inviting sound that pleases your ears, palate, and intellect.

— Withdraw your senses into the middle channel and move Śakti between the two distant poles of Mūlādhāra and Khecarī.

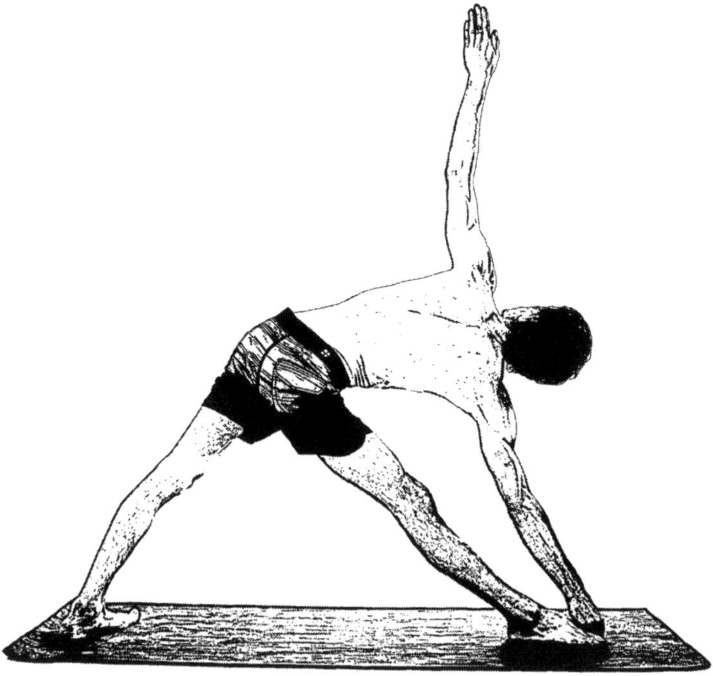

Utthita Trikoṇāsana
(Extended Triangle Pose)

— Rotate your front thigh out so your kneecap faces up.

— Rotate your back thigh out so your kneecap faces to the side.

— Stamp your feet; lengthen your legs; ground your thighs, and anchor your lower body.

— Tip your pelvis to the side; lengthen your spine from tail to head along a horizontal axis.

— Reach up through your top arm with the force of a rocket launching into space.

— Plant your bottom hand; firmly brace the arm.

— Probe space with your spine; make a spiral gesture of extension; open your chest and contemplate infinity.

— Use your immovable bottom arm, and your adamant legs to support the weight of your spine and head.

— Revolve your chest, turn your head, and gaze up past your thumb with ease.

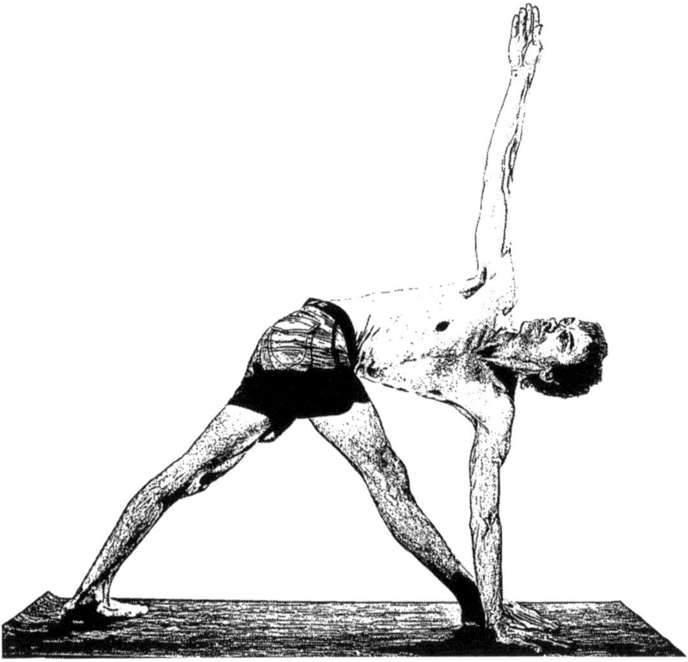

Parivṛtta Trikoṇāsana
(Revolved Triangle Pose)

— Plant your feet and lengthen your legs.

— Ground your thighs and brace your pelvis.

— Rotate your front leg out and your back leg in; scissor your legs together.

— Lengthen your spine from tail to head, and spin your torso along the horizontal axis.

— Line up the joints of your legs and arms as well as your pelvis, torso, and head in the side plane.

— Lengthen both arms; reach vertically up through your top arm while your bottom hand strikes the earth.

— Open your chest to the sky, lengthen your neck; turn your head; gaze up past your thumb.

— Catch Uḍḍīyāna Bandha; rotate your navel; send Prāṇa along your spine from tail to head.

— Light up your five main skeletal lines; awaken your creative fire; take control of your pose; playfully express this sacred Yantra form in your own way.

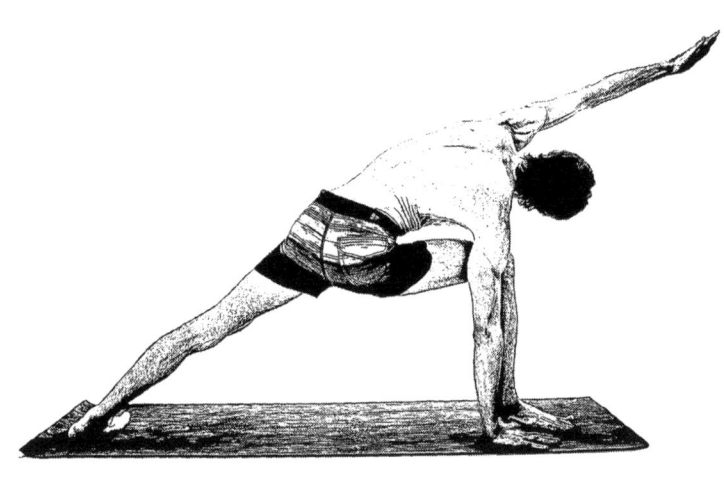

Utthita Pārśvakoṇāsana
(Extended Side Angle Pose)

— Lunge! Make your right thigh parallel to the ground, and stack the knee over the ankle.

— Swing your right knee to meet your right arm.

— Press your right fingertips or hand on the ground, and brace your right arm.

— Reach up through your top arm on the diagonal; line up the arm over your left ear.

— Lengthen your back leg from hip to foot.

— Ground your back thigh; press the femur bone deep into the flesh of the leg.

— Brace the back leg to resist the lunge of your front leg.

— Reach down through your back leg and up through the top arm.

— Your back leg, spine, and top arm form an unbroken diagonal line in the side plane.

— Rotate your spine along the diagonal line; open your chest and navel to the sky.

— Gaze upward from in front of your top arm; then turn your eyeballs in the sockets and gaze at your left palm while continuing to align your head with your torso.

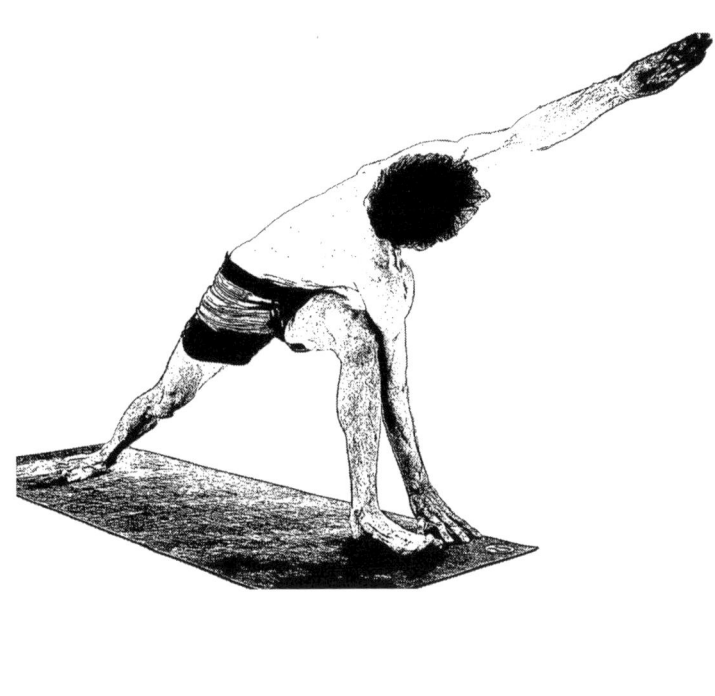

Parivṛtta Pārśvakoṇāsana
(Revolved Side Angle Pose)

— Lunge deeply; drive your front thigh down and forward in the side plane.
— Lift your back heel slightly off the ground.
— Make your front thighbone parallel to the ground.
— Tuck your right buttock; swing your right thigh to meet your firm left arm.
— Be up on the fingertips of your left hand or meet the challenge of pressing your whole hand down without making concessions with other parts of your body.
— Reach up and away through your top arm on the same diagonal line as your back leg.
— Extend your back leg; lift your back thigh without lifting the front hip.
— Work your angled back heel down to the ground in increments while retaining your overall form.
— Lift your head and chest and rotate your spine evenly.
— Line up your top arm and spine along the diagonal line that begins with your back leg.
— Spin; navel and sternum face the sky.
— Gaze up to the sky in front of your top arm.

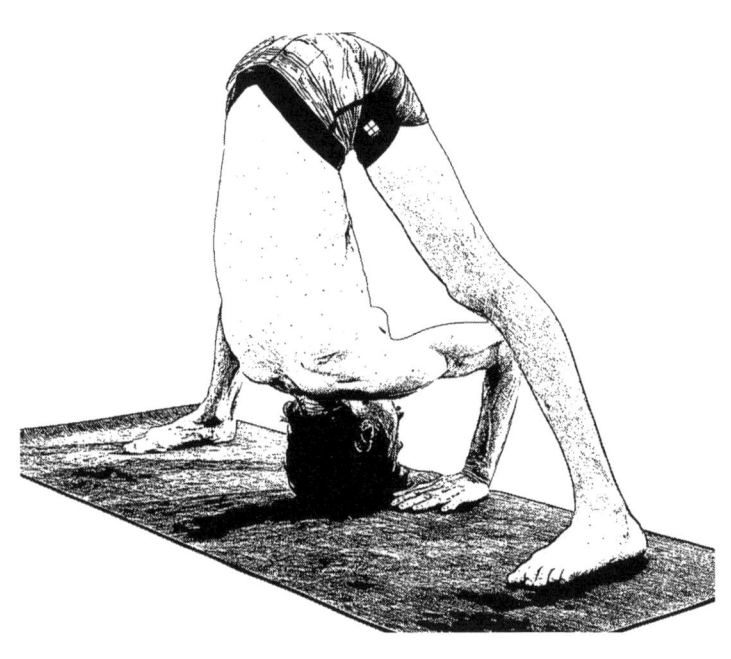

Prasārita Pādottānāsana A

(Wide Legged Intense Forward Bend Pose)

— Adopt a wide stance.
— Root down through the feet; ground the thighs.
— Shift your pelvis forward; plant your head on the ground in line with your feet.
— Walk the hands back; make the upper arm bones parallel to the ground; elbows over the wrists.
— Lift up the pelvis; lengthen the leg bones.
— Embrace being upside down; risk playfully, become immovable on the edge of a precipice.
— Equally ground your head, feet, and hands; five distinct parts plugging into the earth.
— Release your spine from tail to head.
— Broaden your palate and fly your belly up, transform your abdomen into a deep, hollow cave.
— Breathe into your kidneys; fill up your lungs with a mighty expansion.
— Empty your lungs with a contractile force that travels the spine to the pelvic base.

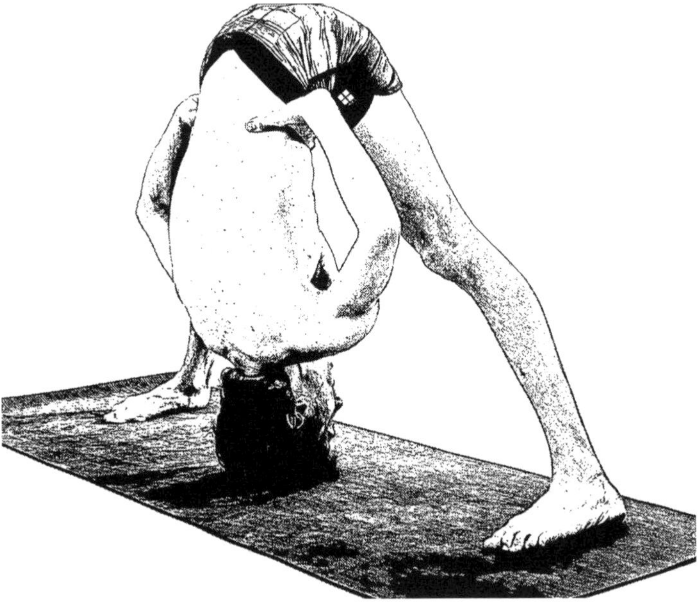

Prasārita Pādottānāsana B

(Wide Legged Intense Forward Bend Pose)

— Wide stance.

— Shift your hips into a vertical line over your knees and ankles.

— Place equal weight upon your head and feet.

— Plant your hands on your waist; use each secret mudrā to subtly stabilize your position.

— Make your legs tall and sturdy; immovable and yielding like the sacred earth.

— Fold at your groin like a ragdoll; release your spine from tail to head.

— Embrace the point of imbalance, become immovable on the edge of a precipice.

— Hollow your abdomen by performing the mudrā Uḍḍīyāna Bandha.

— Wake up your center; tap the creative energy stored at the root of your spine.

— Be at home upside down; travel the axis; make pilgrimages to the 3 sacred caves: your palate, heart center, and sacrum.

— Charge your subtle body with vital energy; cause unwanted thoughts to vanish playfully.

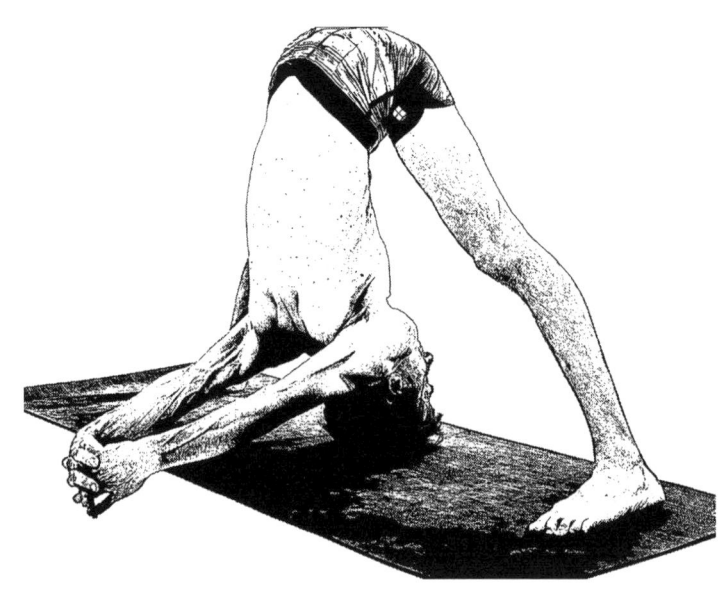

Prasārita Pādottānāsana C
(Wide Legged Intense Forward Bend Pose)

— Wide stance.

— Ground your feet and thighs.

— Plant your head on the ground in line with your feet.

— Reach back through your arms; lengthen the line from your shoulders to your fingers and lower your arms towards the ground.

— Ground your head for leverage to work your arms closer to the ground.

— Inhale and exhale with sound; constrict your throat to control the rhythm, speed, and tone of your breath.

— Remain stubbornly rooted in position; patiently work to open your shoulders.

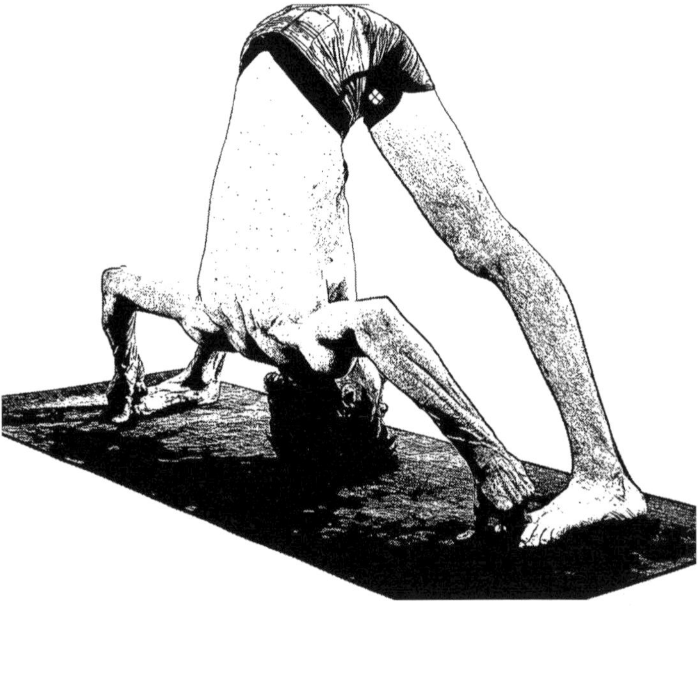

Prasārita Pādottānāsana D

(Wide Legged Intense Forward Bend Pose)

— Wide stance.

— Plant your head on the ground in line with your feet.

— Stamp your feet down; lengthen your leg bones and grow a taller stance.

— Grip your toes with your fingers and brace your arms; make each mudrā count.

— Embrace the inversion; shift forward; play on the edge of imbalance; gain a steady position and deal a blow to your fear.

— Transfer weight into your head, release your spine and round your back.

— Scoop your belly into a hollow without effort.

— Inhale into your kidneys and up to your palate; breathe out along the axis to your pelvic floor.

— Gaze down the nose or to the horizon.

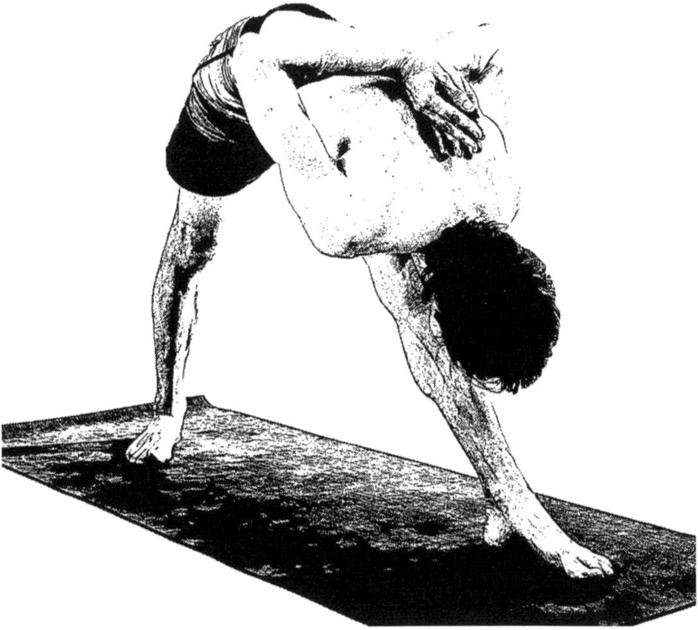

Pārśvottānāsana
(Side Intense Forward Bend Pose)

— Plant your feet, project your hips back and lengthen your legs infinitely.

— Resist from your calf as you lengthen your front leg; avoid pushing your knee back too easily.

— Elongate your spine and rotate your navel to the right.

— Lower your torso towards your grounded front leg.

— Roll back your shoulders, lift your elbows, and brace your arms.

— Press your hands together firmly.

— Go with the downward pull of gravity; deepen the forward bend, drape your torso over your strong legs.

— Drop your forehead or chin onto the shin; bow to the sacred earth.

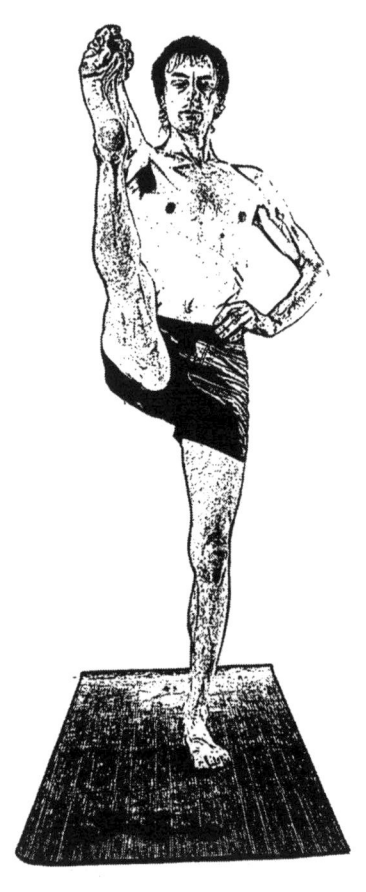

Utthita Hasta Pādāṅguṣṭhāsana
UPRIGHT (Extended Hand to Big Toe Pose)

— Firmly grip your big toe with your fingers.

— Extend your right leg; thrust forward from hip to toes; be patient, seek maximum leg length.

— Pull back with your right arm; resist the forward thrust of your extended leg; refrain from bending your elbow.

— Lift up your right leg to maximum height without sacrificing extension.

— Pull up with your right arm to help lift the leg.

— Vertically align your head, torso, pelvis, and standing leg.

— Know this pose as Samasthitiḥ in disguise; don't be fooled by the added challenge of brilliantly extending one leg.

— Ground your left thigh; suck your navel up and hollow your belly.

— Your left hand grips your waist while your left arm braces.

— Broaden your chest and project your collarbones forward.

— Constrict your throat and breathe with sound.

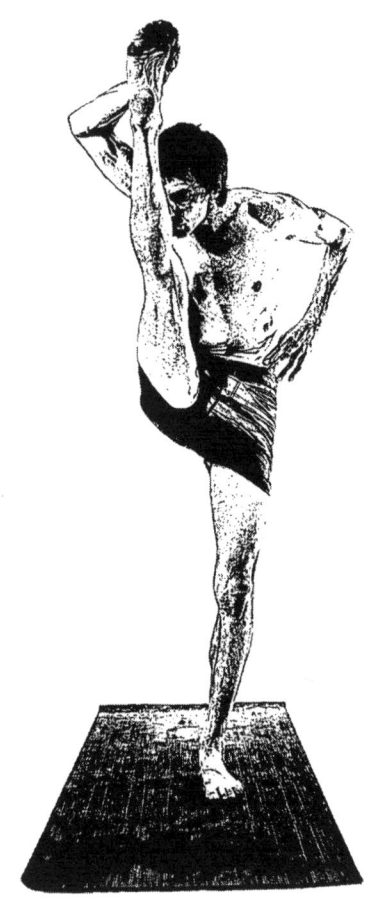

Utthita Hasta Pādāṅguṣṭhāsana
BOWING FORWARD (Extended Hand to Big Toe Pose)

— Kick up strongly with your right leg while at the same time bowing forward.
— Lift your right leg up to meet your body rather than forcing your head down to meet your leg.
— Vigorously pull up with your right arm to help lift up your right leg.
— Stamp your left foot down and ground your left thigh.
— Stabilize your pelvis; hold firm to the axis, avoid shifting your pelvis back as you bow forward and lift your leg.
— Gaze forward with focus and determination.
— Engage yourself entirely in the challenging task; purify and grow strong.

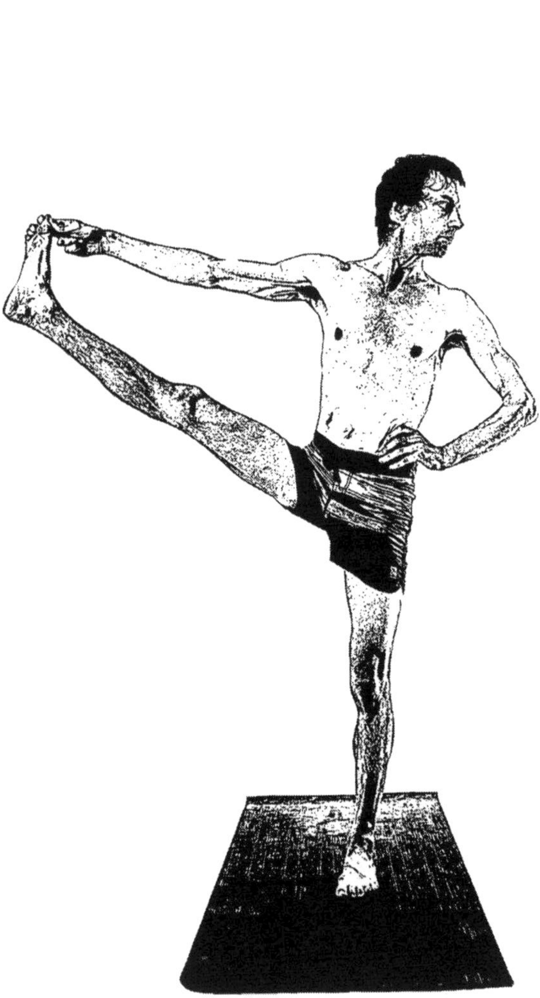

Utthita Hasta Pādāṅguṣṭhāsana

SIDE PLANE (Extended Hand to Big Toe Pose)

— Reach away out to the side through your extended right leg.

— Increase the grip on your big toe and pull towards you with your right arm without bending your elbow.

— Lean slightly to the left and root down through your left leg.

— Firmly grip your waist with the left hand and stabilize your left arm.

— Lift up your navel and sternum, turn your head to the left, and cast a steady gaze to the side.

— Remain steady in position for any amount of time; win skill in balance and strengthen your will.

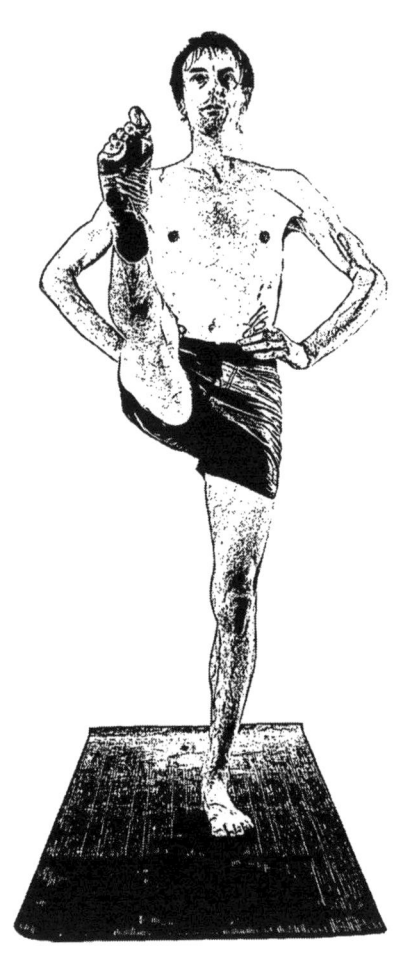

Utthita Hasta Pādāṅguṣṭhāsana
HANDS AT WAIST (Extended Hand to Big Toe Pose)

— Kick forward and up through your right leg like a Kung Fu master.
— Your head, torso, pelvis, and left leg form a stable, vertical column.
— Ground your left thigh; pull up from the root of your spine.
— Lift up your belly and expand your chest.
— Pull down with your hands to lift up your chest.
— Project your collarbones forward and lift your right leg.
— Gaze forward towards the horizon to steady your balance.
— Will your body to remain steady in this upright position and transform your vertical axis into an unbreakable Pillar of Fire.
— Embrace the tapas; steady your limbs, eyes, ears and palate; gain the fruit of Indriya Jaya (mastery of your senses).

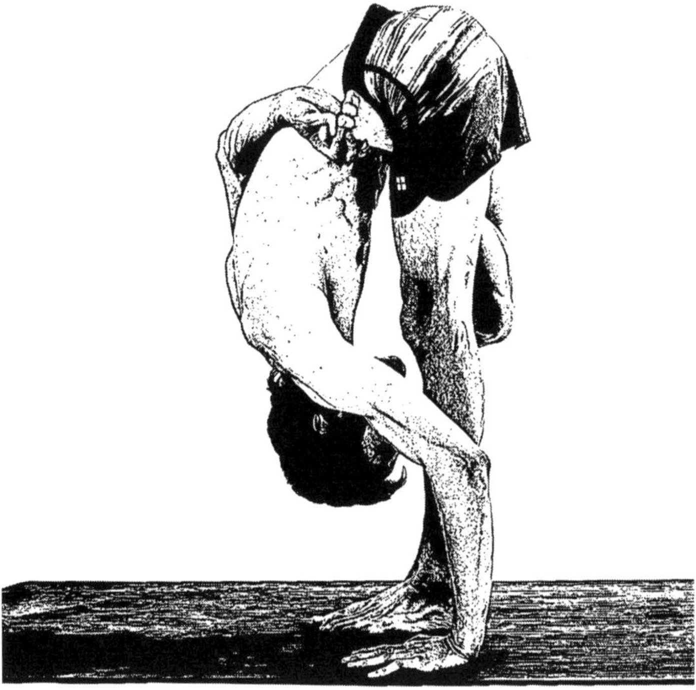

Ardha Baddha Padmottānāsana
(Half Bound Lotus Stretching Pose)

— Balance on your tall standing leg, the main weight bearer of your pose.

— Vertically line up your hip, knee, and ankle.

— Stabilize your left calf and press your thighbone back; extend your leg infinitely.

— Plant your left hand firmly beside your left foot and brace your left arm.

— Release your head downward, free your spine, and love being inverted on the edge of imbalance.

— Slowly move your head and torso towards your grounded standing leg.

— Square your hips; press your lotus leg back until your knee reaches the side plane; then brace.

— Press your right heal up into your belly; trigger Uḍḍīyāna Bandha (belly flying up gesture).

— Firmly grip your right foot with your right hand; seal in energy; every mudrā stabilizes your pose.

— Gaze towards your shin.

— Breathe with sound up and down the axis.

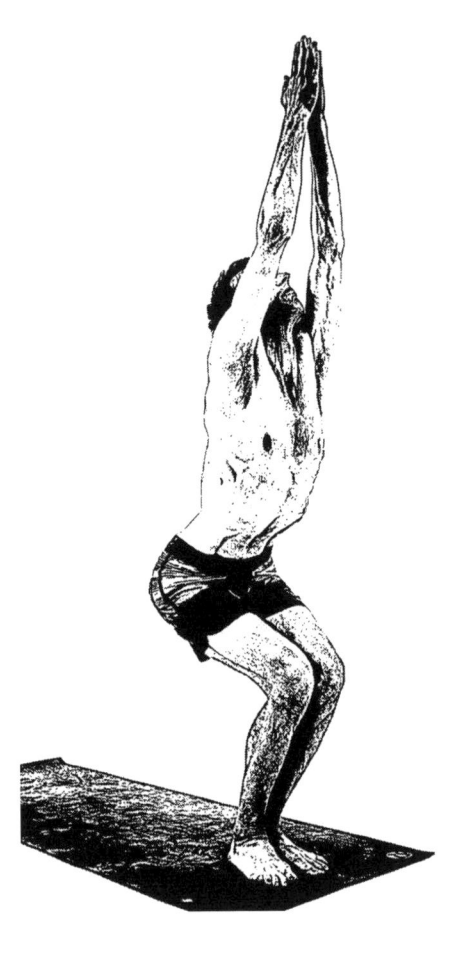

Utkaṭāsana
(Fierce Pose)

— Drive your knees and thighs forward and lower your pelvis vertically toward your heels.

— Shift your whole body forward.

— Weight the balls of the feet more than the heels; achieve a deep lunge, an accurate half squat.

— Reach your arms up on a diagonal line that is just forward of the vertical axis.

— Shoot your arms diagonally up towards the sky like a rocket headed into space.

— Weight your tailbone, pull up your navel, and level your pelvis on the same diagonal line as your spine/arms.

— Expand your armpit chest and project your upper spine forward.

— Draw your front ribs down and widen your back ribs.

— Pull up forcefully from the Mūlādhāra at the base of your spine and cause awakened Śakti to fly up the middle channel.

— Transform your body into a lightning bolt, a dynamic zigzag shape made of 3 main lines; your shins, thighs, and spine/arms.

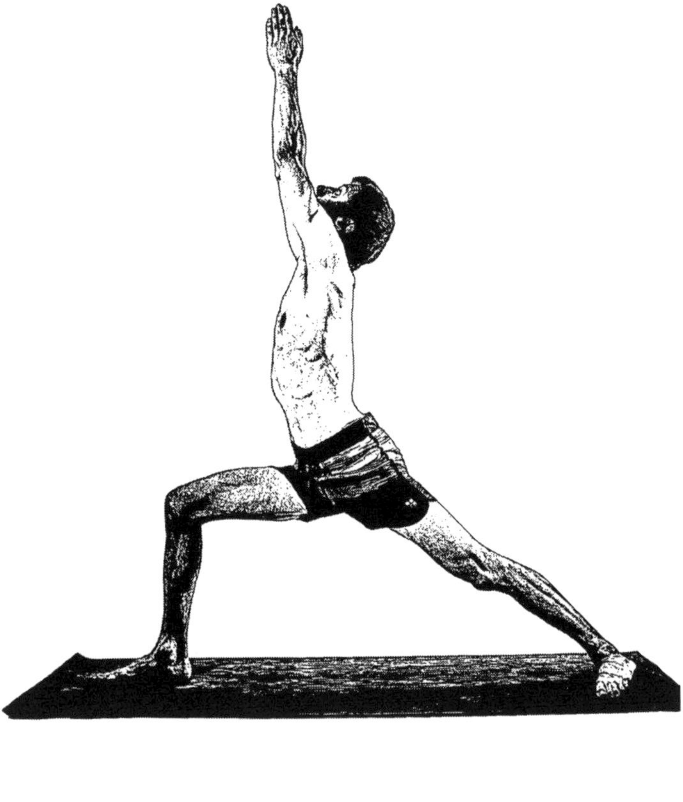

Vīrabhadrāsana A
(Warrior Pose)

— Drive your right thigh forward into a deep lunge.

— Track your right thigh in a line from the hip to the knee; line up the knee over the ankle.

— Swing your left hip forward towards square and extend the back leg from hip to foot.

— Lift up your navel and weight your tailbone; bring your pelvis towards level and lessen any anterior tilt.

— Widen the back ribs; broaden the mid torso; suck the lower front ribs down.

— Lift your chest; project your collarbones forward; line up the top of your sternum directly over the bottom of your sternum.

— Shoot your arms vertically up to the sky; reach up with the power of a rocket launching into space.

— Square your shoulders and trunk.

— Take your head back and gaze up past the thumbs while retaining length through the back of your neck.

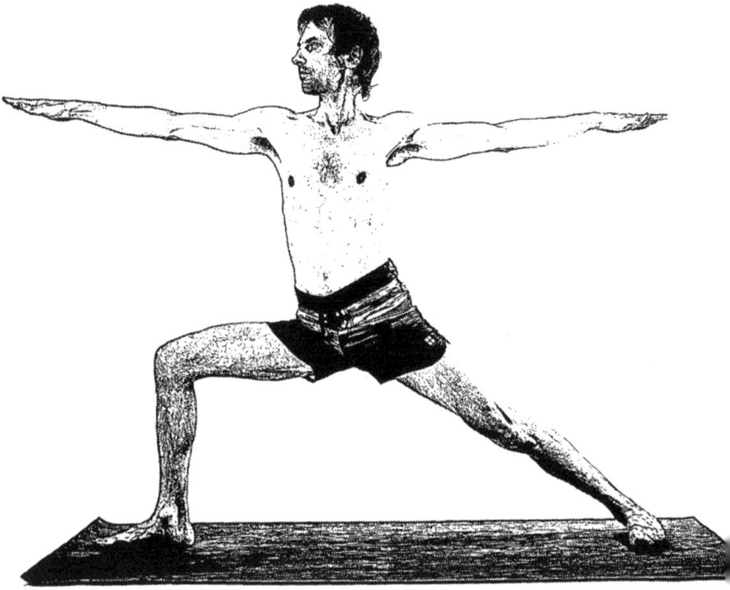

Vīrabhadrāsana B

(Warrior Pose)

— Lunge; make your right thigh parallel to the ground and line up your knee over your ankle.

— Externally rotate your front hip; swing your right knee to the right; release your outer right hip toward the ground.

— Externally rotate the back hip; make the kneecap face forward.

— Stamp your back foot down and extend your back leg.

— Your thighbones are the weight bearers of your pose.

— Pull up the navel and lengthen your coccyx; create a neutral pelvic base.

— Lift up from the root of your pelvis; grow your spine vertically upward and expand your chest.

— Contemplate the infinite by pulling into your back arm and reaching your arms horizontally away from each other.

— Gaze past your right fingers in the side plane.

— Charge your legs, arms, and spine with intelligence and vitality; adjust your pose by moving energy inside your body; behold as the sacred form is revealed.

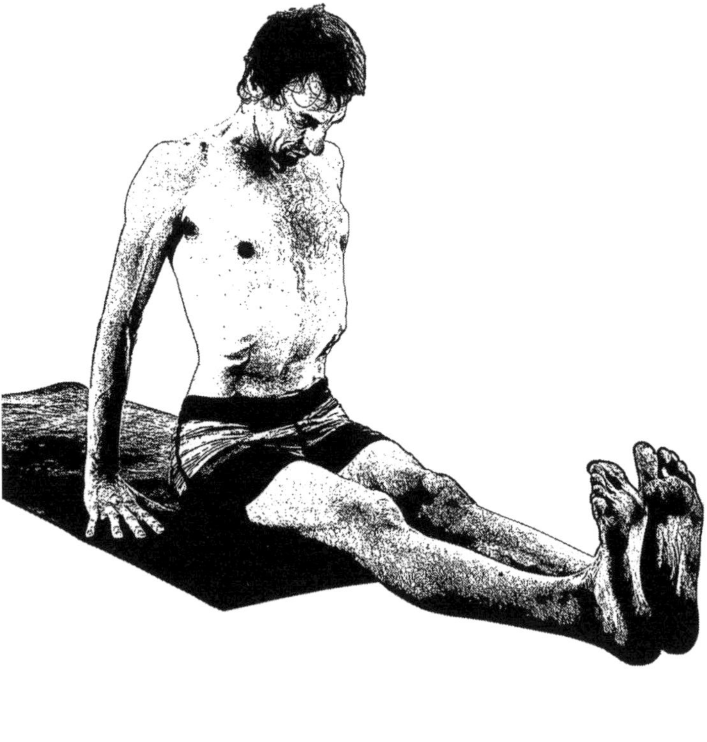

Daṇḍāsana
(Staff Pose)

— Sit forward on your sitting bones, extend your legs brilliantly and stamp the femur bones down.

— Make your legs into levers; long, strong sticks that tether you to the earth and free your spine.

— Weight your tail and lift up your belly from the root.

— Level your pelvis and grow your spine tall along the vertical axis.

— Broaden your chest; roll your shoulder heads into the side plane.

— Widen your kidneys and suck your front lower ribs down and back towards your spine.

— Plant your fingertips beside (and behind) the pelvis; firm your arms and legs in unison.

— Open your chest and bow the forehead.

— Lock your chin to the rising chest and seal in vital energy from above.

— Weight your whole body and awaken the root; raise Śakti and watch energy rocket up the main channel.

— Transform the middle axis into a Pillar of Fire; enter this glorious channel through absorption; burn up all perceptions, and become void-minded.

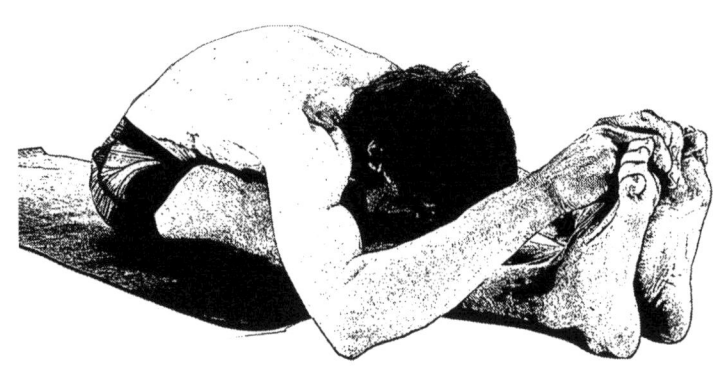

Paścimatānāsana A

(Intense Western Stretching Pose)

— Root down your thighs and brilliantly extend your legs.

— Firmly grip your big toes with your middle and index fingers.

— Push your feet away and brace your arms with your elbows lifted.

— Strengthen your legs and arms; wake up the muscles; make your limbs dense, compact, inert, and yet alive with creative expression.

— Stop your limbs; fix their position; store up earth power.

— Lengthen your spine; come down to your legs and to the earth.

— Pull up your navel; lift your belly; wake up your spine from the root.

— Plant your head on your shins and release your trunk onto your anchored legs.

— Gaze forward or down; release your neck.

— Constrict the throat and breathe with sound.

— Direct the flow of your breath up and down the axis; send the expansion force of your inhalation upward from the pelvic floor to the heart center; send the contraction force of your exhalation downward from the heart center to the pelvic floor.

— Draw Śakti up the middle channel.

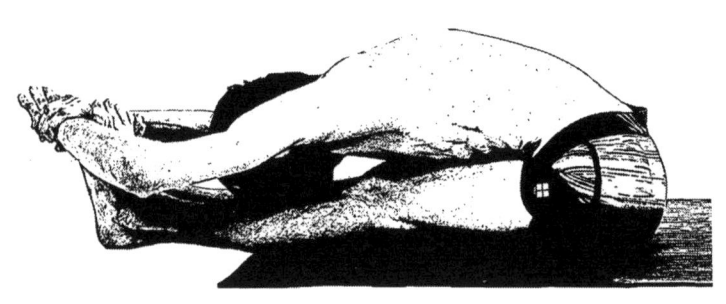

Paścimatānāsana B
(Intense Western Stretching Pose)

— Weight your lower body, stamp your thighs down, fasten your legs to the earth.
— Extend your legs; create infinite reach through the bones from hips to toes.
— Hover your torso above your legs and lengthen; project your spine maximally forward.
— Bring your head to your shins; release your trunk down towards your weighted legs.
— Brace your arms with the elbows lifted.
— Push your feet into your arms and resist with your arms.
— Gaze forward or down; release your neck.
— Breathe into your kidneys; expand the backside of your torso as you fill up your lungs.
— Sweep your exhalation down the length of your spine from your palate to your pelvic floor
— Cause awakened Prāṇa to travel up the backside of your body; visualize the energy flowing from your heels, up the backs of your legs, up the backside of your torso, to the back of your skull. By this means, bow to the sacred western direction and be purified of your past unskillful actions.

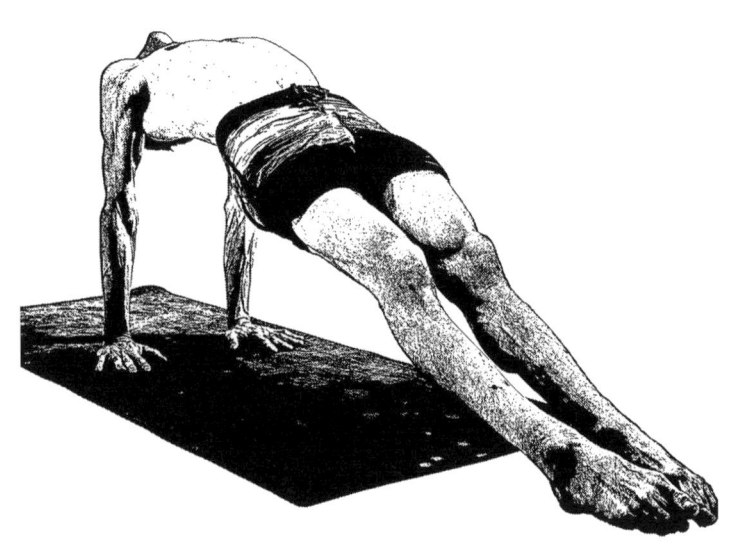

Pūrvatānāsana
(Intense Eastern Stretching Pose)

— Stamp your hands down into the earth, fully extend your arms, and lift your chest into a high dome shape.

— Lengthen your legs with determination; extend the lines from your hips to your toes without letting up.

— Ground your thighs; press the long shafts of the bones deeper into your legs.

— Root your feet into the ground, lift up your sacrum, and suck your spine up into your torso.

— Pull up the pit of your abdomen; draw energy up the axis until your heart blooms.

— Take your head back freely in an arcing circle.

— Reach back through your skull; look down and back along the ground towards your feet.

— Know this pose as Plank in disguise—the root of all strength; stay up in position, perform tapas, strengthen your body and mind.

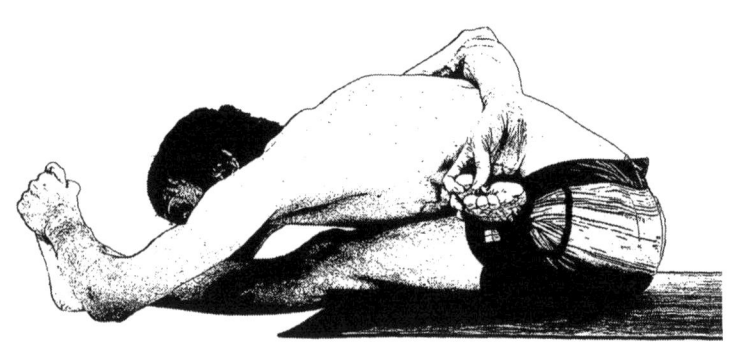

Ardha Baddha Padma Paścimatānāsana

(Half Bound Lotus Western Stretching Pose)

— Root down through your thighs and extend your left leg.

— Firmly grip your feet with your hands.

— Gently pull back on your stable left foot with your left arm for leverage to lengthen your spine.

— Rotate your spine to the left; shift your navel to the left; lay yourself out over your extended leg.

— Press your right heel up into your belly; trigger Uḍḍīyāna Bandha; cause the great bird of Prāṇa to fly in the middle channel without fatigue.

— Release the weight of your whole body; lower down towards the ground and become still; know the sacredness of inertia and discover meditation.

— Lengthen your left leg from hip to toes; lengthen your spine from the base to the crown; perform these actions continuously to contemplate the infinite and merge your mind with the vast, empty sky.

— Gaze forward or down; release your neck and let energy flow freely to your brain and senses.

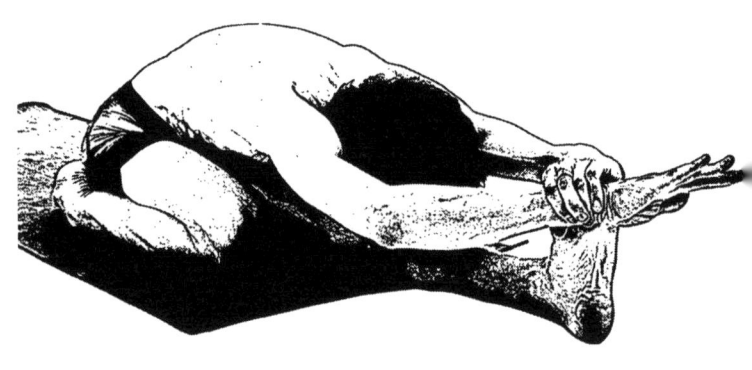

Tiryaṅ Mukhaikapāda Paścimatānāsana

(Three Face One Leg Western Stretching Pose)

— Ground your thighs evenly, press down through your inner left leg.

— Remain centered as you bend forward.

— Firmly grip your right wrist with your left hand around the ball of your left foot.

— Extend your left leg and push your left foot into your interlocked hands; brace your arms, resist the actions of your extended leg and gain leverage to lengthen your spine.

— Accept gravity's downward pull on you; release your body masses to the ground and meet the earth as a friend.

— Internalize the sound of your breath; find a breathing rhythm that penetrates your body; draw vital energy up from the root of your spine and invite Śakti to flow freely within the middle channel.

— Gaze forward with steady eyes, open your inner ears, awaken your palate, and internalize each sense organ.

— Perceive the rhythm of your breath, pump life force into the central Nadi, and experience the world anew.

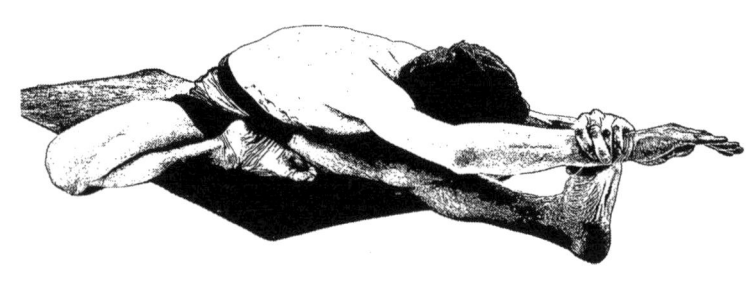

Jānu Śīrṣāsana A
(Head to Knee Pose)

— Root down through your legs; ground your femurs; the earth is your ally.

— Elongate your spine, rotate your navel to the left, and lay out over your extended leg.

— Lengthen your left leg and push your left foot against your stable arms in a play of opposing forces.

— Go with the downward flow of gravity, let your weight come down onto your leg; strike the immovable spot and arrest your mind.

— Drop your forehead down onto your shin; use the strong contact between your head and leg to seal vital energy inside your body.

— Inhale up the backside of your torso and send healing Prāṇa to the adrenal glands on your kidneys.

— Exhale down the length of your spine and send Prāṇa to the root support at your base.

— Gaze forward or down; relax your brain.

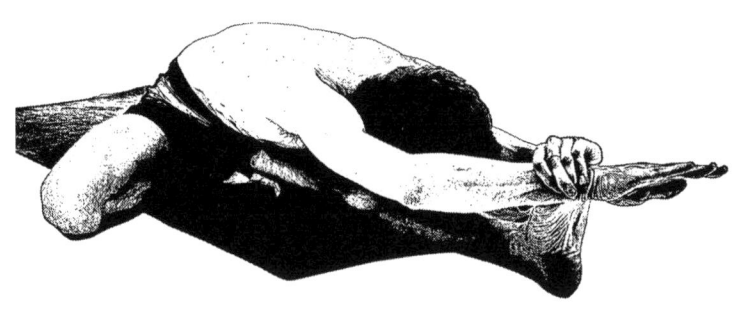

Jānu Śīrṣāsana B
(Head to Knee Pose)

— Ground your legs and pelvis equally.

— Elongate and release your spine.

— Press the pelvic floor with your heel; wake up Mūlādhāra Cakra; tap the source of all energy.

— Extend your left leg continuously as a contemplation of the infinite.

— Push the left toe mounds into the interlocked arms and pull towards you with your arms.

— Plant your head onto your shin; release your weight onto your leg.

— Breathe up and down the length of your spine with the purpose of controlling Śakti inside your body.

— Wake up to the primal rhythm of your breath and make energy flow in the inner circuits; alchemy!

— Perform actions playfully and breath skillfully to make your āsana a sacred geometrical form, a device for absorption.

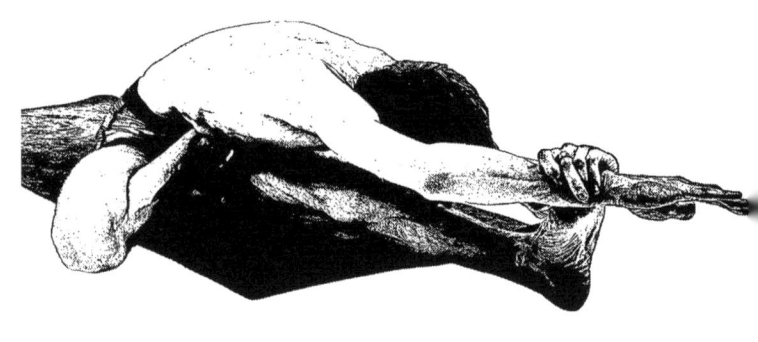

Jānu Śīrṣāsana C
(Head to Knee Pose)

— Angle your right knee and thigh inward to 45 degrees; face your right toes directly to the side.

— Elongate and release your spine; create a deep forward bend and a steady mind.

— Grip your right wrist with your left hand around your left foot; pull back through your arms and find mudrā power.

— Lean slightly to the right and actively press your right toes into the ground.

— Push your foot into the interlocked arms and pull back towards you through your arms.

— Release your head onto the leg; create a potent energetic seal.

— Press your heel into your belly; trigger Uḍḍīyāna Bandha; move Śakti up the axis.

— Strike an unwavering gaze; use your astute ears to follow the illusive sound of your breath; master your sense organs and be visited by equanimity.

— Breathe into your right toes; observe sensation rather than react; view a sweet or bitter taste impartially; gain great merit.

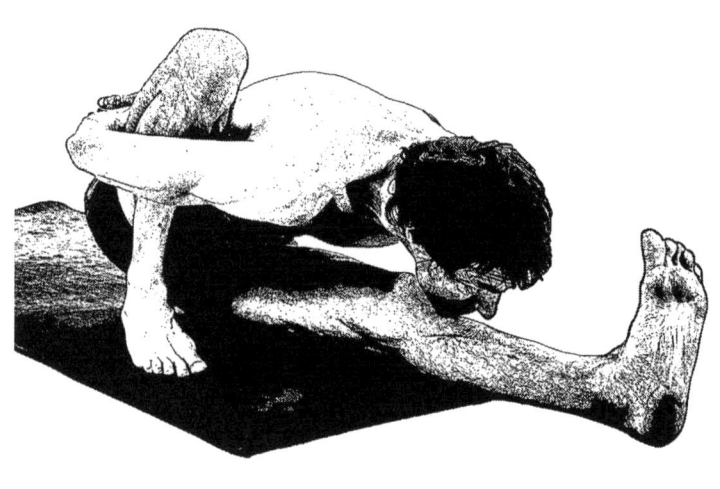

Marīcyāsana A
(Great Sage Pose)

— Stamp your squatting foot down and anchor your left thigh.
— Shift forward, lighten your seat and lift your right sitting bone.
— Project the spine forward and reach back through the arms with the elbows bent.
— Squeeze your squatting leg with your arms.
— Firmly clasp your fingers or grip your left wrist with your right hand.
— Square your hips and shoulders.
— Increase the weight of your spine and head, and come down to your extended leg.
— Gaze forward or down and actively stamp your head onto your shin.
— Exhale down to Mūlādhāra and inhale up to Khecarī; wake up Śakti and light the inner cosmos.
— Each action is a device that seals in vital energy; performing all actions in unison leads you into an ecstatic trance.

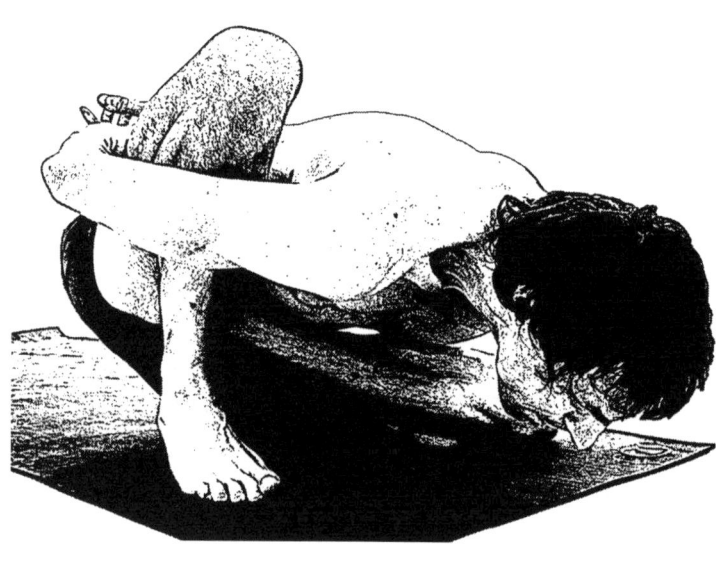

Marīcyāsana B
(Great Sage Pose)

— Shift forward, lift your right sitting bone, and stamp your right foot down into the earth.

— Elongate and release your spine.

— Hug your squatting leg with your arms and create a firm grip with your fingertips or your right hand around your left wrist.

— Square your shoulders and hips; reach forward through your head, project your spine out into space in front of your fixed leg foundation.

— Gaze forward or down without wavering.

— Soften your eyes, ears, palate; use each sense organ to perceive the subtle workings inside your body.

— Follow the contraction force of your exhalation down the axis to its end and galvanize your center.

— Follow the expansion force of your inhalation up the axis; awaken your palate and find the mudrā known as Khecarī, the Space Maker Seal.

— Fill up and empty your lungs thoroughly and follow your breath to the ends of the axis at opposite poles; be a connoisseur of mudrās.

— Stop all movement as a game; know holy inertia and gain Absorption (Samādhi) playfully.

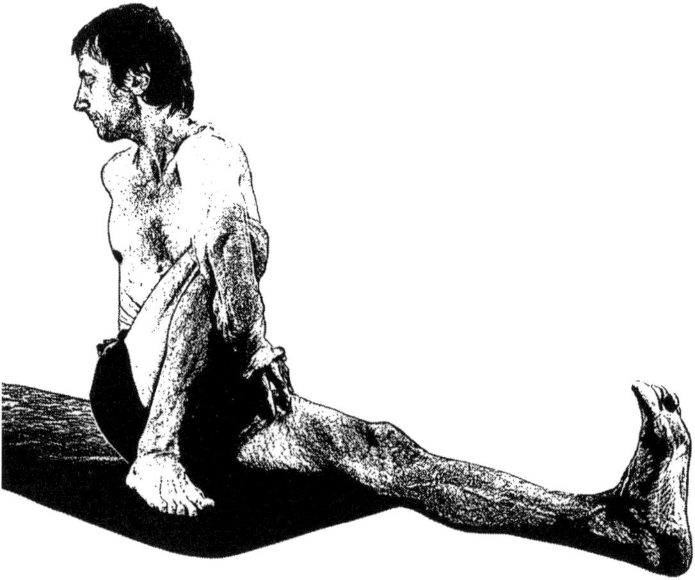

Marīcyāsana C
(Great Sage Pose)

— Shift forward, lift the right sitting bone, and weight your legs.

— Strike down through the squatting foot and ground the thighbone of your extended leg.

— Make your left leg long and strong; a lever that provides grounding force for you to twist.

— Lift up your spine and spin to the right.

— Hug your arms to the squatting leg; brace the leg against the arm pressure.

— Suck your left kidney up and into your body, lift up the right side of your chest and roll back your right shoulder.

— Rotate your spine evenly from base to crown.

— Circle to the right with your eyes; look around to the side and draw your spine into a deeper twist.

— Eyes and nose lead the twist, your spine follows while your legs stubbornly root down into the earth; the combination of actions sets your core ablaze.

— Twist and awaken Kuṇḍalinī; catapult your mind to the secret world inside of you.

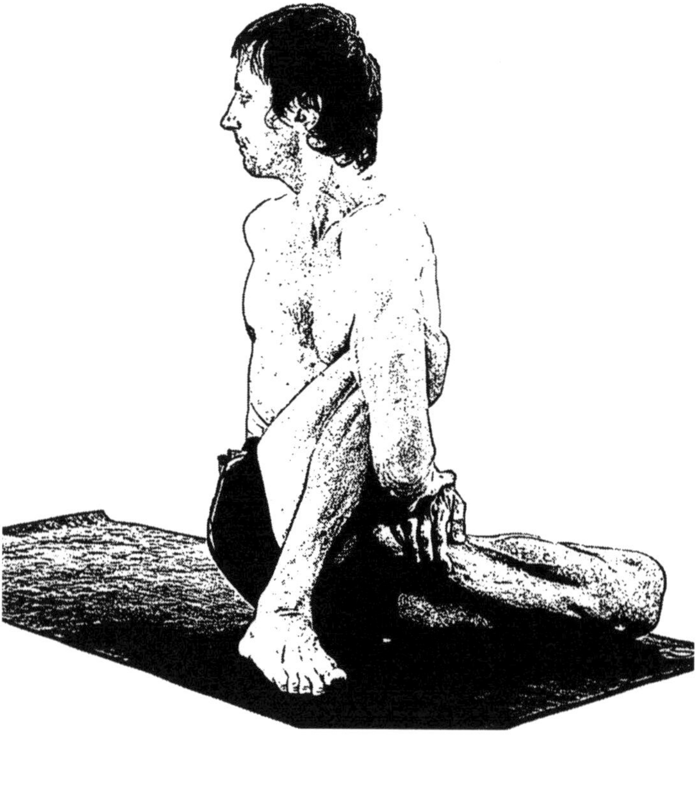

Marīcyāsana D
(Great Sage Pose)

— Shift forward, lift the right sitting bone, and ground your legs.
— Stamp the earth with your right foot; lengthen your left thigh and bring your left knee to the ground.
— Lift up your head and spin to the right.
— Wrap your arms snugly around your right leg and firmly connect your hands.
— Internally rotate your arms; palms face out.
— Squeeze your right leg with your arms for leverage to increase the spinal twist.
— Lift up your spine from the root and rotate evenly along the axis from the base upward.
— Suck your left kidney up and into your torso, lift the right side of your chest, and roll back your right shoulder.
— Circle to the right with your eyes; get your whole body involved in the rotation.
— Free your breath any amount; breathe in or out a bit more.
— Twist; awaken the vital energy at your base and draw life force up the middle channel; delight in moving Śakti inside your body.

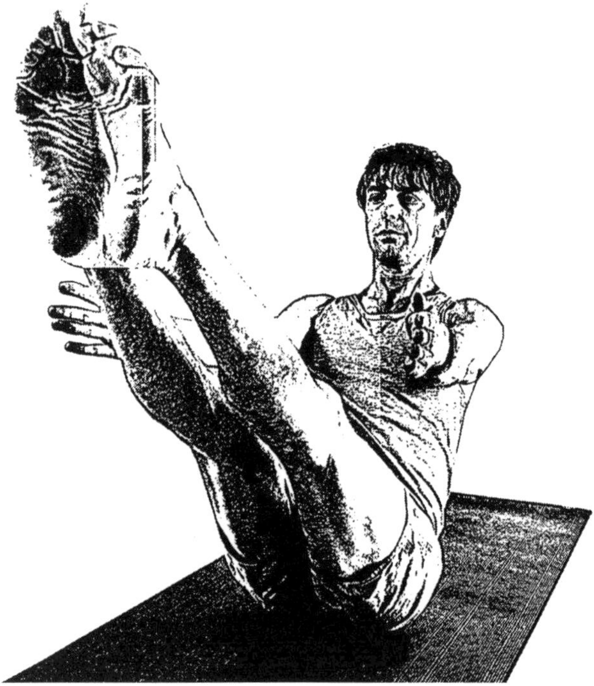

Nāvāsana

(Boat Pose)

— Lift your chest and feet equally; your eyes in a horizontal line with your feet.

— Stay forward on your sitting bones and stabilize your seat.

— Lean your upper body back, slightly curl your upper spine into flexion and yet project your sternum forward.

— Kick your feet up and away from you; brilliantly extend your legs with the force of a rocket launching into space.

— Reach horizontally forward through your arms from shoulders to fingertips for leverage to lean back through your upper body.

— Suck up your navel; hollow your abdomen; lengthen rather than harden your belly muscles.

— Circle your inhalation behind your belly; breathe into your back ribs and kidneys.

— Cast a steady gaze forward.

— Focus on the three main lines of your boat pose: 1. pelvis/torso/head line 2. legs line 3. arms line. Send powerful laser beams of awakened energy shooting out through these lines as you stay firmly rooted in position.

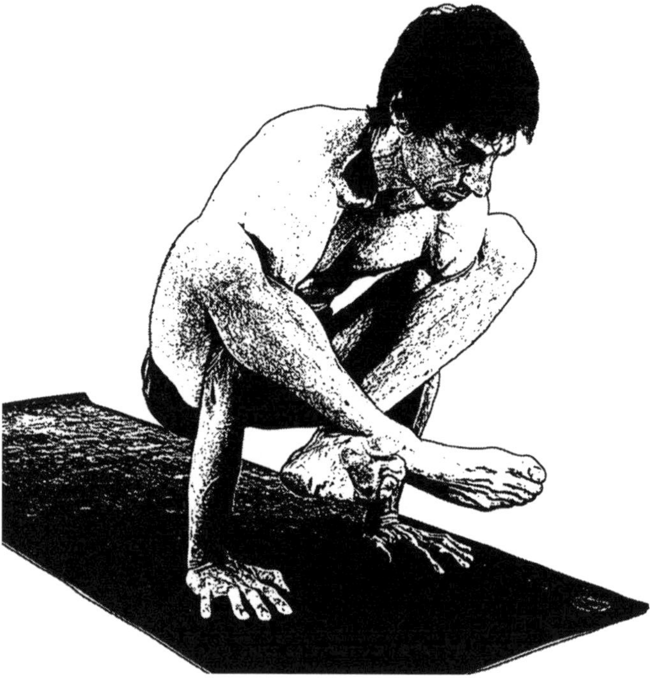

Bhuja-Pīḍāsana
UPRIGHT POSITION (Arm Pressure Pose)

— Ground your hands and make your arms strong like twin tree trunks; easily rest your torso and legs on this adamant support.

— Keep your torso upright, your feet lifted, and your pelvis sunk down towards the ground.

— Squeeze your arms with your legs and snug together your crossed ankles.

— Extend your arms infinitely and lift away from the earth.

— Withdraw your senses to the central axis deep within your torso and locate your diaphragm muscle; control its piston like action and breathe in and out more thoroughly.

— Cast a steady gaze downward or forward or upward.

— Know this root arm balance position as a unique meditation seat and remain steady in an agreeable position without fatigue.

— Use your stay to learn how actions relate to each other; swiftly arrange your skeleton into your desired geometrical configuration; unify your body to unify your consciousness.

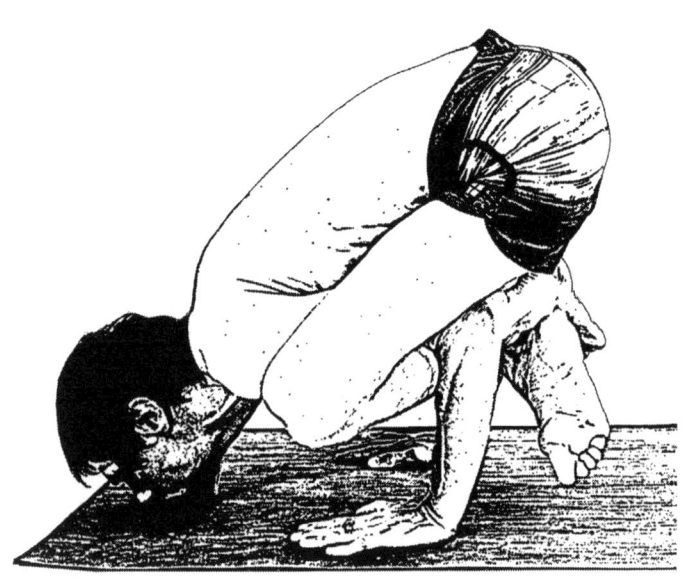

Bhuja-Pīḍāsana
FORWARD BEND (Arm Pressure Pose)

— Keep your hips shifted back and weight your arms more than your head.

— Stamp down with your hands and strengthen your arms.

— Hover in a low position balancing on your arms with your head either off or on the ground.

— Lightly stamp your forehead or chin on the ground and pull up your feet and shins without lifting your pelvis.

— Steady your gaze; focus on a point forward or down; gaze as a device to steady your body and mind.

— Play as you hover in position; know the point of greatest stability is found on the edge of imbalance; bow to the earth, free your breath and clear the field of you mind.

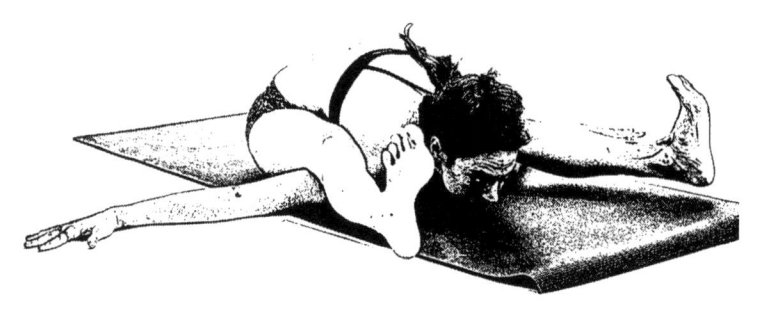

Kūrmāsana

(Tortoise Pose)

— Push forward through your heels and extend your legs.

— Bring your head to the ground and lengthen your spine.

— Lengthen your arms out to the sides away from each other.

— Brace your arms and stamp down through your hands.

— Increase your weight; go with the benevolent force of gravity; ground your entire body and connect to the earth; know the sacred healer.

— Withdraw your attention from outside to inside; internalize your gaze and be at home inside your body.

— Control Prāṇa by controlling the primal expansion and contraction rhythm of your breath.

— Channel your energy; send revitalizing energy up and down your spine; wake up the subtle circuits throughout your body; reverse aging and keep death away.

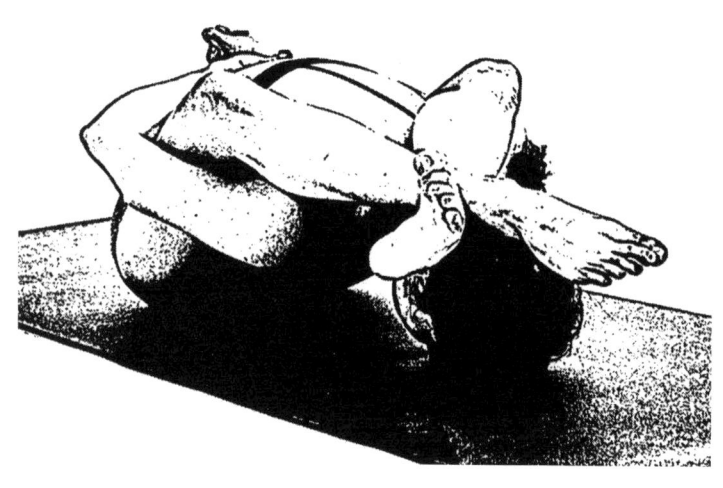

Supta-Kūrmāsana
(Laying Down Tortoise Pose)

— Root down through your hips and weight your head.

— Snug your crossed ankles to each other.

— Externally rotate your femurs within the hip sockets and stabilize your legs.

— Clasp your fingers and brace your arms.

— Allow your spine to round in flexion.

— Subtly nudge your head forward to elongate your spine.

— Allow your body to release and go with the downward pull of gravity.

— Imitate a tortoise and withdraw into your shell; seek solitude, refuge, and protection.

— Know this Yantra is a sacred form for bowing to the earth and practicing Pratyāhāra, recovering your senses.

— Visit the cave of your palate and open your inner ears; discover your breath's internal mantra, So Ham, I Am That.

— Gaze within your heart center; quest for a vision.

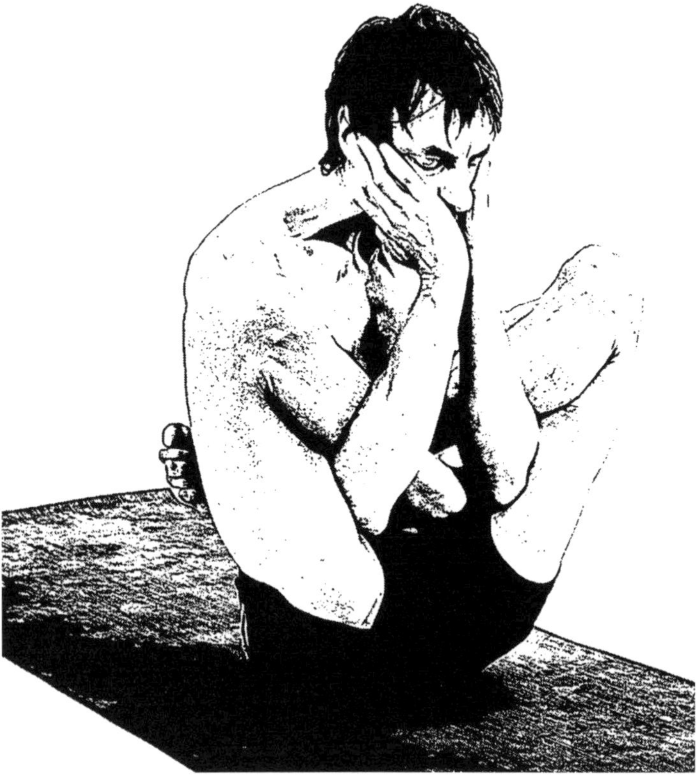

Garbha Piṇḍāsana
(Embryo in the Womb Pose)

— Bow your head, increase the connection between your hands and chin.

— Push your chin down into your hands and lift up your head and chest.

— Draw your knees closer together and suck your thighs to your chest.

— Stabilize your compact shape on the edge of imbalance.

— Gaze downward and withdraw your senses to the core of your body.

— Regulate the piston like action of your diaphragm; send this large sheet-like muscle down and up to fill and empty your lungs.

— Work your breath pump and control the flow of energy in your body.

— Take charge of each action and seal in energy with each mudrā; reveal the secret source of energy that drives your posture and your efforts.

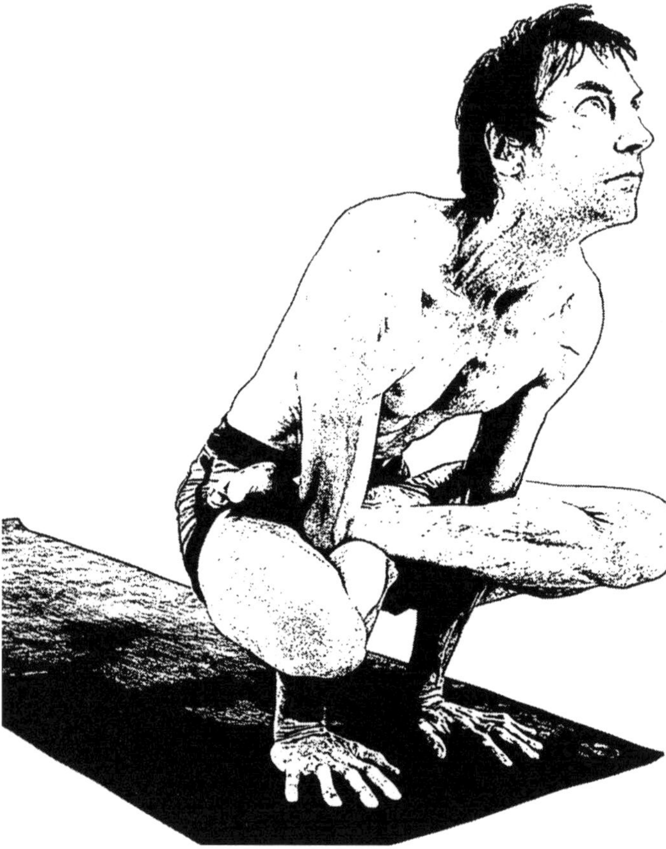

Kukkuṭāsana
(Rooster Pose)

— Root your hands and lift up your legs.
— Boldly shift forward; strike a confident pose in the risk zone; dexterously play with the edge of imbalance.
— Imagine your arms are like twin tree trunks with roots deep in the earth that anchor you in position.
— Suck your knees towards each other.
— Increase the snug bind of your legs in Lotus.
— Equally lift up your hips and thighs.
— Look up with a receptive gaze that matches the vast open sky.
— Exhale down the middle channel; awaken the energy at the root of your spine.
— Inhale up the middle channel; draw the Śakti up to your heart center and palate.
— Transform your sacrum, heart center, and palate into three sacred caves along the axis; attain powers like grounding at will or creating space inside your body whenever you choose.

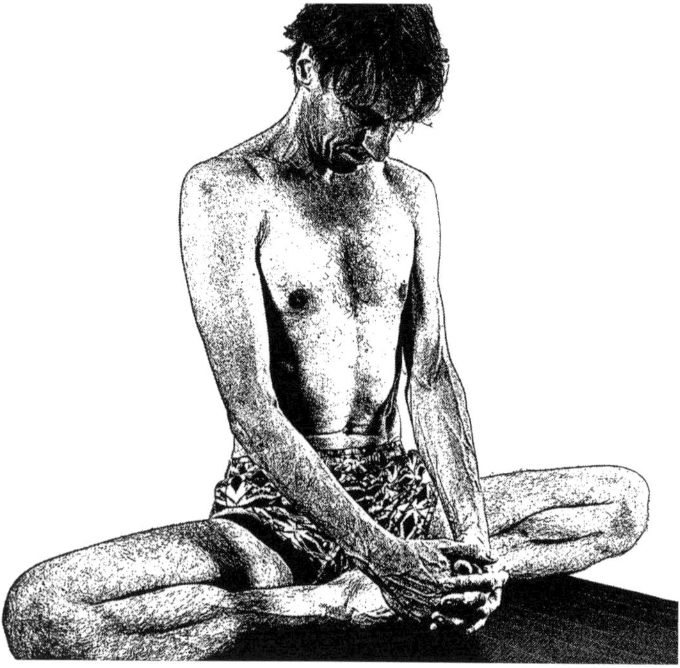

Baddha Koṇāsana
UPRIGHT POSITION (Bound Angle Pose)

— Sit on your sitting bones with a neutral pelvis.

— Vertically align your head, torso, and pelvis.

— Root down through your thighs and create an immovable seat.

— Clasp your fingers around your toes; pull up with your hands and brace your arms.

— Press your heels together and lengthen your thighbones away from each other.

— Send laser beams of awakened energy flowing through the long shafts of your femur bones from hips to knees.

— Fly your belly up into a deep hollow and lift your chest into a mighty expansion.

— Lower your chin to meet your rising chest.

— Gently press your tongue against the roots of your upper teeth.

— Awaken your palate and the power of Khecarī Mudrā, The Space Maker Seal.

— When you exhale, send the centripetal force called Apāna Vāyu down to the root of your spine.

— When you inhale, send the centrifugal force called Prāṇa Vāyu up to the root of your palate.

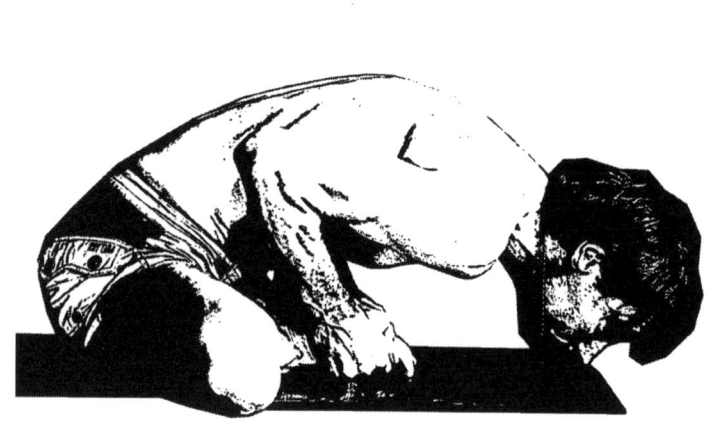

Baddha Koṇāsana
FORWARD BEND (Bound Angle Pose)

— Anchor your pelvis and stamp down into the earth with your thighbones.

— Launch away from your grounded legs; project your head and chest forward; daringly reach out into space with your spine.

— Use the strength of your backbone to hover with control just above the ground.

— Surrender your weight to the ground; bow down to the earth, with astute presence of mind.

— Lengthen your thighbones; direct life force through the bones from hips to knees.

— Exhale with an aspirant Ham sound and inhale with a sibilant So sound; listen to the internal mantra that spontaneously arises with each breath you take.

— Make pilgrimages to the sacred caves of Mūlādhāra (sacrum), Anāhata (heart center), and Khecarī (palate), and become absorbed in Suṣumnā (the central axis).

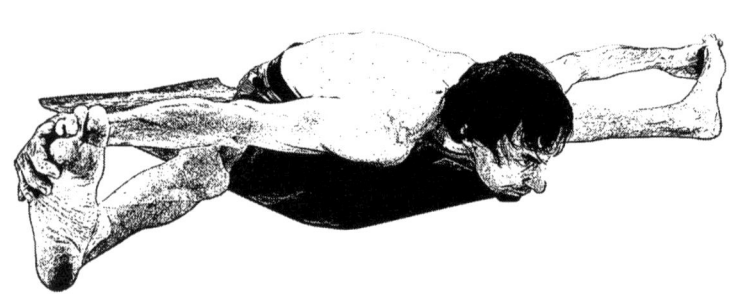

Upaviṣṭa Koṇāsana
VARIATION A (Seated Angle Pose)

— Anchor your lower body; weight your pelvis; stamp down your thighs.

— Project your feet away; lengthen your legs.

— Pull back through your arms and resist the mighty forward reach of your legs.

— Project your torso forward; boldly reach your spine out into space and hover just above the ground with control.

— Skillfully surrender your weight to the earth; bring your chin, chest, and navel to the ground with poise.

— Gaze upwards towards the energy center between your eyebrows (Ajna).

— Find absorption in the great swinging rhythm of your breath.

— Direct the sound of your breath through your legs, arms, and along the central channel.

— Breathe and move Śakti inside your body with poise, skill, playfulness, and abandon.

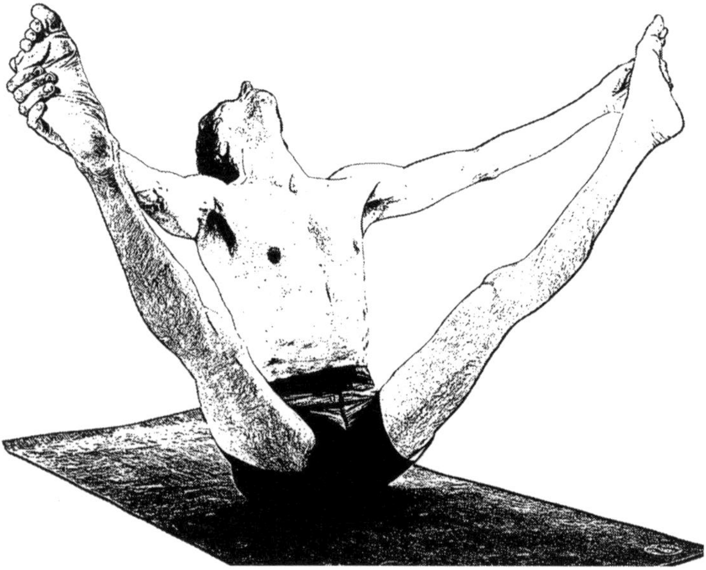

Upaviṣṭa Koṇāsana
VARIATION B (Seated Angle Pose)

— Balance in mid-air on the edge of imbalance; fearless.

— Grip your outer feet with your hands and extend your legs vigorously forward.

— Pull back towards you through your arms to resist the forward thrust of your legs.

— Keep your arms extended as you pull back against the forward driving force of your legs.

— Use the opposing actions of your limbs to ride forward onto your sitting bones and stabilize your seat.

— Lean your upper body back and lift your chest into a mighty expansion.

— Reach up and over with your head; draw a confident circle across the sky with your nose.

— Awaken your center by playing with the push and pull forces passing through your legs and arms.

— Cause Prāṇa to spring up from the base and light up the famous energy centers along the glorious axis.

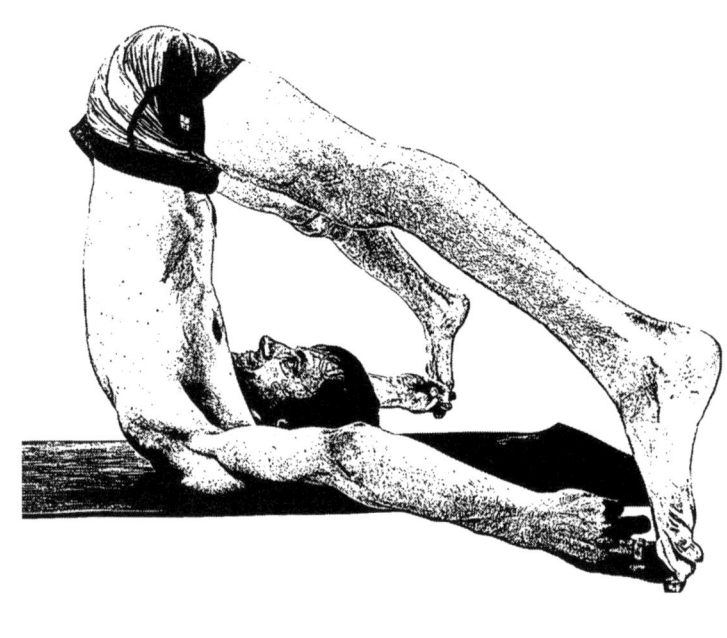

Supta Koṇāsana
(Laying Down Angle Pose)

— Grip your big toes with your fingers; extend your arms and legs.
— Reach away through your legs and pull back towards you with your fully extended arms.
— Lift up your hips and make your spine taller.
— Lift your sitting bones and inner thighs.
— Lock your chin to your chest and perform the worthy gesture called Jālandhara Bandha.
— Exhale along the central axis to the base of your spine and suck your abdomen into a hollow.
— Look up the front of your body and view Mūlādhāra Cakra, the prized root support lotus.
— Imagine lines of awakened energy emanating from your center and charging through your legs, arms, and spine; lengthen these energy lines as a device to contemplate the infinite and wake up the higher faculty of your mind.

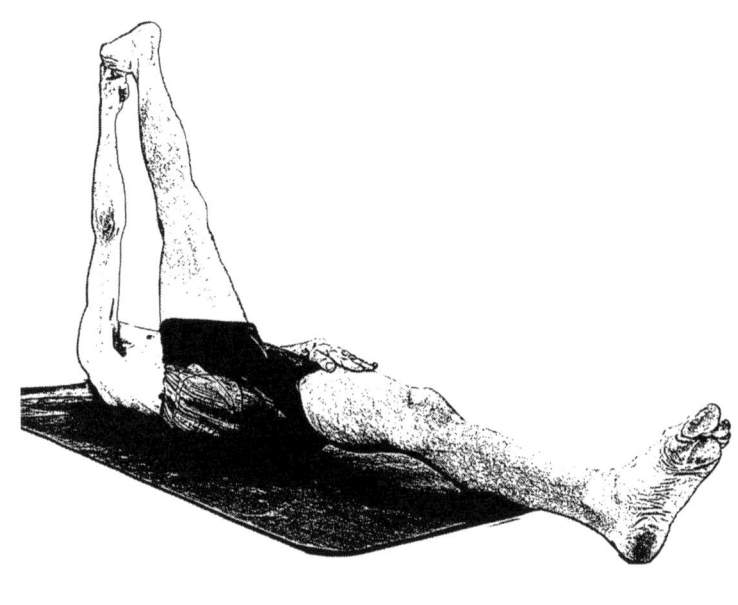
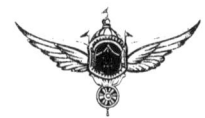

Supta Pādāṅguṣṭhāsana

SET-UP POSITION (Laying Down Hand to Big Toe Posture)

— Use the ground beneath you as a horizontal plane to line up your head, torso, pelvis, and left leg.

— Brilliantly extend your right leg; thrust upwards through the bones from hip to toes.

— Grip your right toe, strengthen your right arm, and pull your right leg down towards you.

— Stamp your left hand down onto your left thigh.

— Lengthen your tailbone and pull up your navel.

— Keep your sacrum flat on the ground and widen your back ribs.

— Widen your collarbones and suck your front lower ribs down and in towards your spine.

— Keep your chin level and gaze along your lifted leg.

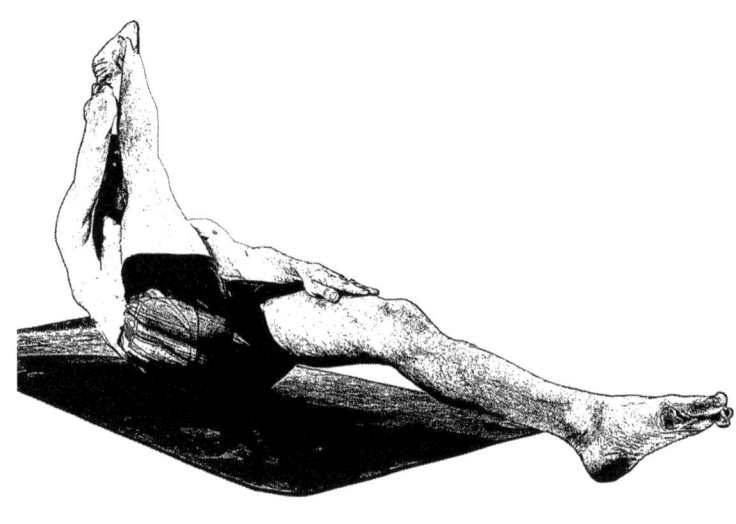

Supta Pādāṅguṣṭhāsana
LIFT BODY UP POSITION
 (Laying Down Hand to Big Toe Posture)

— Grip your right big toe firmly and lift up your torso away from the earth with a mighty surge of power.

— Lengthen and strengthen your right leg and brace your right arm.

— Touch your chin or forehead to your shin and then lift the unit of your right leg and head/torso further away from the ground.

— Extend your left leg and ground the right thigh.

— Extend your left arm and stamp your left hand down onto your left thigh.

— Engage your belly muscles by your effort to lift your torso away from the ground.

— Scan through your limbs and spine; extract work from every part of your body.

— Find pure effort; engage yourself entirely in expressing this formidable Yantra.

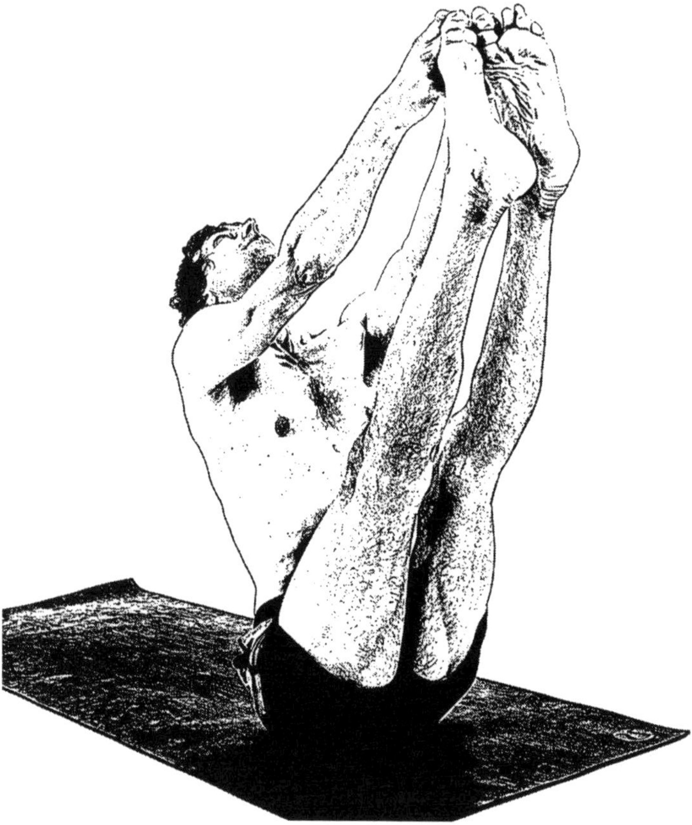

Ubhaya Pādāṅguṣṭhāsana
(Both Big Toes Pose)

— Boldly stop your body in midair; become stable on the edge of imbalance.
— Kick forward with your feet and strengthen your grip on your toes.
— Powerfully extend your legs and pull back through your arms to resist the forward thrust of your legs.
— Lean back through your upper body and ride forward on your sitting bones.
— Keep your arms brilliantly extended; lengthen and strengthen the line that spans from your shoulders to your fingers.
— Lift up your navel and widen your chest.
— Take your head back with a confident throw; look up and over with a circular gaze.
— Control your diaphragm; play with the expansion and contraction rhythm of your breath; cause healing energy to flow freely throughout your body.

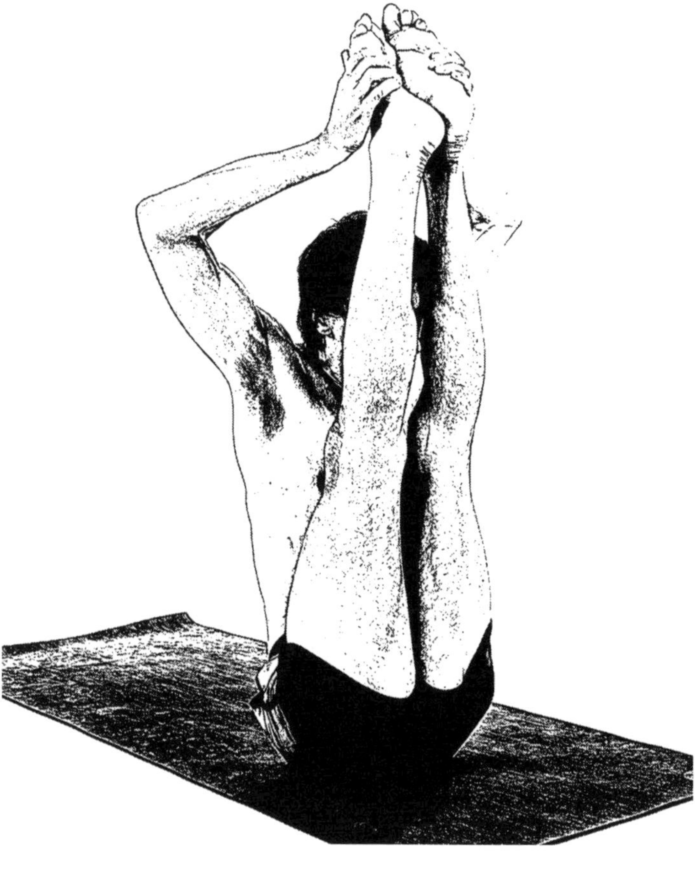

Ūrdhva Mukha Paścimattānāsana

(Upward Facing Western Stretch Pose)

— Reach up through your legs in a gesture of brilliant extension and pull down firmly on your feet with your hands.

— Lift up your chest, navel, and draw your torso closer to your strong, unmoving legs.

— Plant your forehead onto your shins; bend your elbows out to the sides and brace your arms.

— Shift forward towards your sitting bones and create a super stable position on the edge of imbalance.

— Gaze along your shins or up towards your feet.

— Allow this super charged version of Paścimattānāsana to teach you that dynamism transforms the dross of inertia into the gold of awakened consciousness.

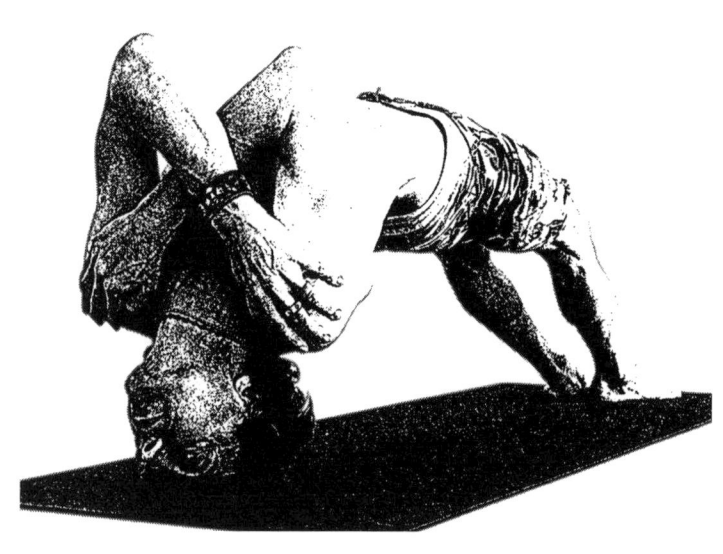

Setu Bandhāsana
(Bridge Pose)

— Dome your chest and suck your entire spine higher up into your torso.

— Ground your head; hook your fingers firmly above your collarbones and pull down through your crossed arms from fingers to elbows.

— Root down through your feet and brilliantly extend your legs.

— Draw your sacrum up into your body and hollow your belling into Uḍḍīyāna Bandha (Belly Flying Up Gesture).

— Subtly shift from the top of your head towards your forehead.

— Gaze down your nose or between your eyebrows.

— Activate your arms and legs to create a strong support structure and activate your spine to create a strong arch.

— With great vigor and determination, transform your whole body into a shapely, indestructible bridge.

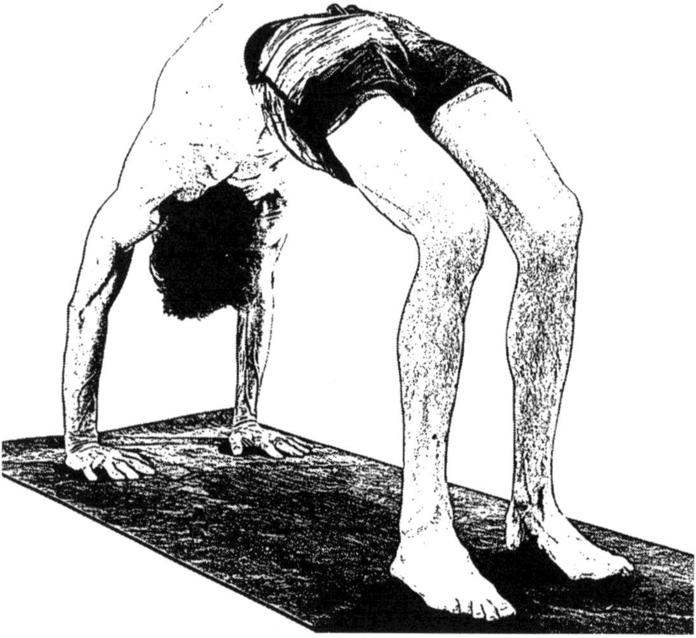

Ūrdhva Dhanurāsana
(Upward Bow Pose)

— Press down through your hands and feet.

— Extend your arms, lift up your torso, and project your arched spine away from the ground.

— Subtly shift your weight into your legs and vertically line up your knees over your ankles.

— Draw your knees towards each other, release your inner thighs, and fix your legs in position.

— Subtly shift your weight into your arms; work to vertically stack your shoulders, elbows, and wrists; suck your upper spine forward and open your chest.

— Center your body equally between your hands and feet and equally weight your arms and legs.

— Maximize the height of your belly and achieve the tallest possible rainbow arch; lift your navel up to the celestial realms and cause the Gods and Goddesses to marvel.

— Take your head down and back in contrast to sucking your spine up and forward.

— Pull up the navel and send the inhalation up into your chest.

— Anchor your limbs and pull up the mighty force of Śakti from the root of your spine; achieve skill in back bending and win the power to move mountains.

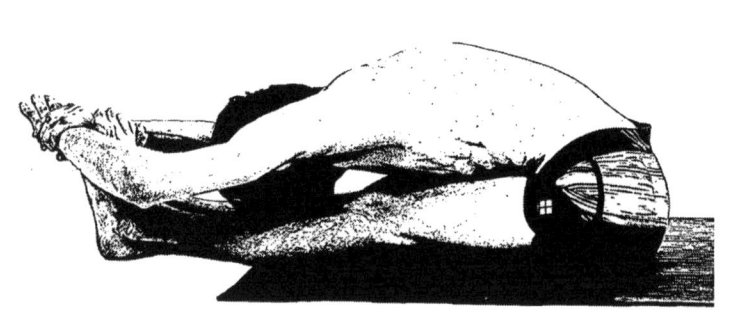

Paścimattānāsana
(Intense Western Stretching Pose)

— Root down through your thighs and lengthen your legs.
— Project your torso forward and release your body down onto your legs.
— Push away through your feet and pull back through your arms.
— Suck your navel forward and lengthen your spine from the base.
— Plant your chin or forehead onto your shins and clear the field of your mind.
— Gaze downwards at a point along your legs or more forward towards your feet.
— Breathe into the backside of your body, massage your kidneys with the flow of your breath, send healing Prāṇa, awakened energy, to your adrenal glands on top of your kidneys, and calm your nervous system and sense organs.

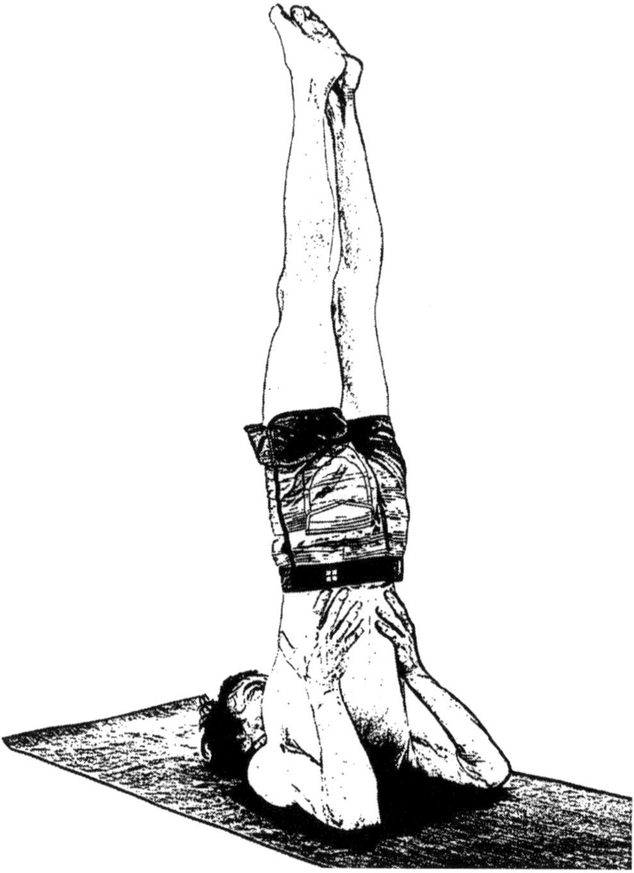

Sālamba Sarvāṅgāsana
(All Limbs Pose)

— Vertically stack your ankles, knees, hips, and shoulders.

— Broaden your chest and project your spine and pelvis forward to the vertical plumb line.

— Push your hands forward into your back and project your torso back into your hands while continuing to open your chest.

— Brace your arms; form your fingers and palms into a strong basket that catches and supports your weight.

— Shoot your legs up to the sky with great force and lessen the burden of weight on your arms.

— Press your thighbones back; lodge the shaft of the thigh bones deep into the flesh of your legs.

— Perform Jālandhara Bandha; lift your chest to meet your chin; release your throat.

— Gaze up the front of your body to adjust your pose; galvanize the forces of your limb levers and light up the spinal axis with your inspired tapas.

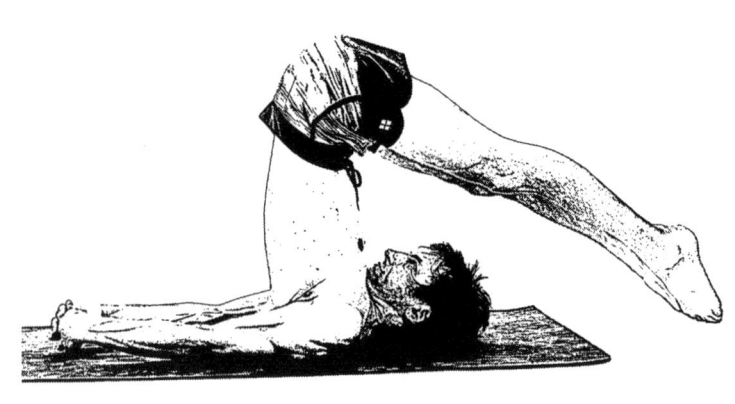

Halāsana
(Plow Pose)

— Lift up your pelvis and extend your legs and arms.
— Line up the hips vertically over your shoulders.
— Root down through your arms from shoulders to fingers.
— Extend your legs with vigor and press your toes into the ground.
— Charge your leg muscles with vitality; make the flesh dense, compact, inert, and yet awake with intelligence.
— Elevate your sitting bones and lift up your inner thighs.
— Widen your collarbones and lock your chin onto your chest.
— Gaze up the front of your body and withdraw your mind to the interior; use your other eyes to see the sacred magic within the physical form.
— Let the oceanic ebb and flow rhythm of your breath come alive within you.
— Send mighty forces whirling through your legs, arms, and spine.

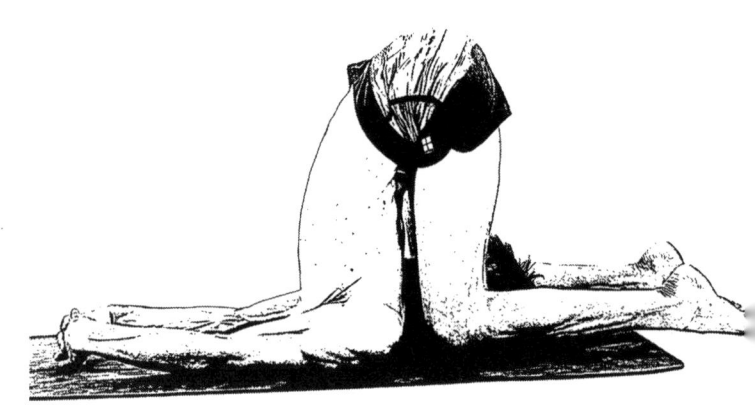

Karṇa Pīḍāsana
(Ear Pressure Pose)

— Shift back towards your shoulders and take pressure off of your neck.

— Lengthen your arms from shoulders to fingers and root them down into the ground.

— Squeeze your ears with your inner knees and brace your legs.

— Increase the weight of your legs and arms; stabilize your pelvis along the vertical axis to maintain the integrity of your form as your limbs come down closer to the ground.

— Practice Pratyāhāra; squeeze your ears with your knees and become absorbed in the flow of your breath; listen to the great sound.

— Strike an immovable spot, create inward absorption, and find the magical world inside your body.

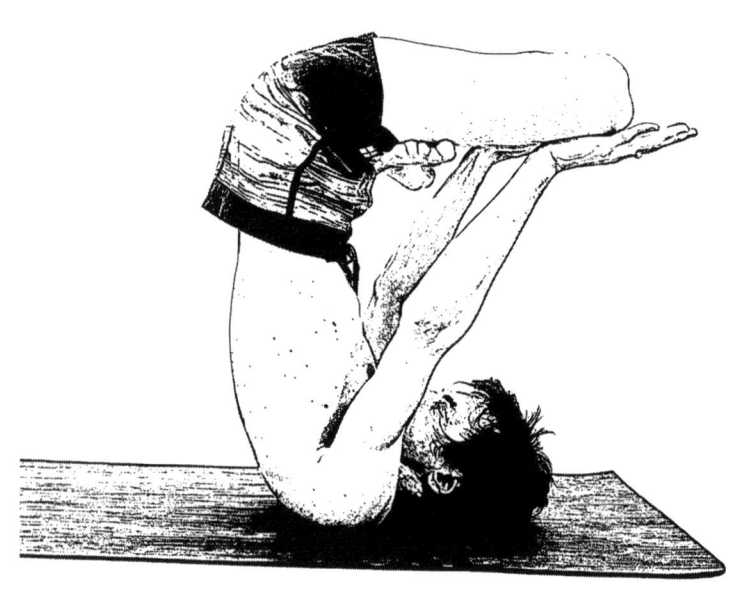

Ūrdhva Padmāsana

(Inverted Lotus Pose)

— Push up through your arms and press down through your legs.

— Fully extend your arms and make your thighs parallel to the ground.

— Line up the pelvis vertically over your shoulders and make your spine tall.

— Press your hands into your knees and your knees into your hands to suck your abdomen into a deep hollow.

— Subtly shift back and weight your shoulders instead of your neck, and yet increase the weight passing through your arms and legs.

— Use this dicey meditation seat to know that the point of greatest stability is found on the edge of imbalance.

— Lift your chest to meet your chin and perform Jālandhara Bandha (Chin Lock).

— Cast a connoisseur's gaze up the front of your body to the root of your pelvis; wake up the creative energy sleeping within Mūlādhāra, your root cakra.

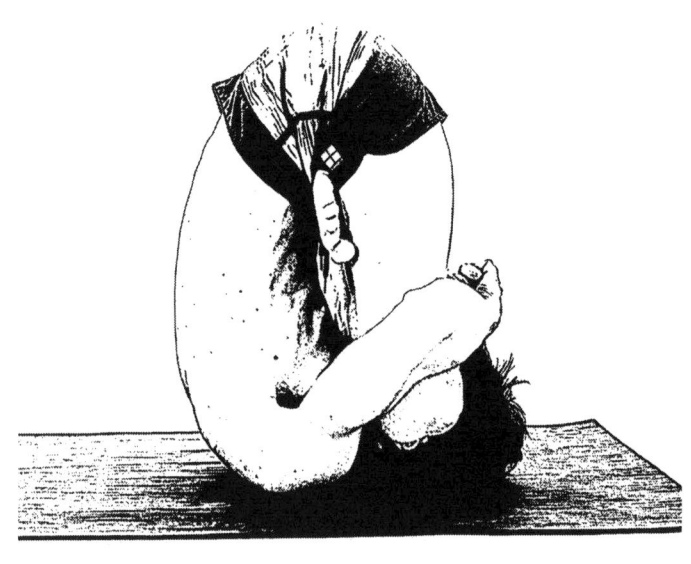

Piṇḍāsana
(Embryo Pose)

— Shift weight onto your upper back and off of your neck.

— Squeeze your bound legs with your arms like a sailor tying a favorite knot.

— Draw your legs towards your body and increase the compactness of your shape.

— Stabilize your pelvis in subtle opposition to lowering your knees towards the ground.

— Balance with ease and view this odd inversion as simply another glorious meditation seat.

— Listen to the smooth sound of your breath and empty your mind of unwanted thoughts.

— Place your senses in the cave of your heart and perceive the world from there; taste medicine that heals.

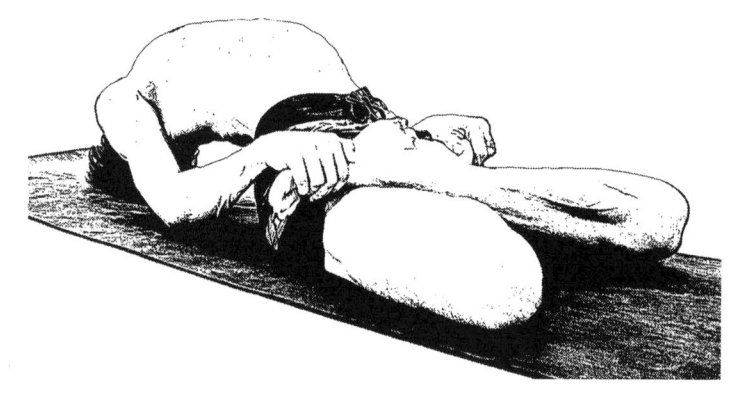

Matsyāsana
(Fish Pose)

— Lift up your chest into a high dome shape.
— Ground your legs and root your pelvis.
— Suck your knees towards each other; brace your arms with your elbows up off the ground.
— Pull back on your feet with your hands.
— Ground your head and coil your upper spine into a neat curve within your chest.
— Lift the pit of your abdomen, send your inhalation up the axis, and expand your chest to a marvelous extent.
— Gaze between your eyebrows.
— Awaken energy at the base of your spine; send Prāṇa up to your heart center and then to your palate; accomplish the feat of moving Śakti inside your own body; become deserving of success and evade death playfully.

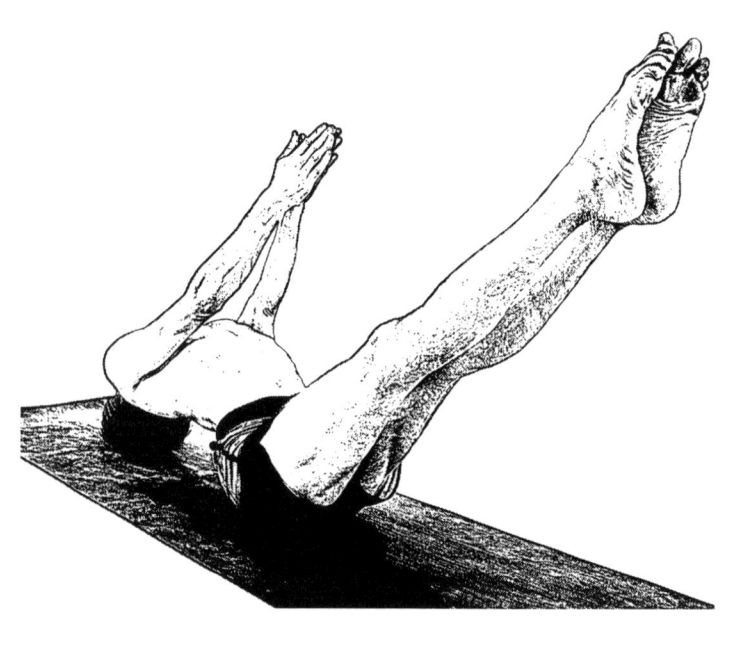

Uttāna Pādāsana

(Extended Legs Pose)

— Lift up your chest and suck your spine into a deep arch within your torso.

— Ground your head and root your pelvis.

— Reach up and away on parallel diagonal lines through your arms and legs.

— Send laser beams of awakened energy shooting up through your legs from hips to toes and through your arms from shoulders to fingers.

— Use the force of your diagonal arm reach to lift your chest into a high dome shape.

— Pull up your navel and perform the belly flying up gesture (Uḍḍīyāna Bandha) to open your heart center.

— Cast a circular gaze back and down towards the ground or look down your nose.

— Train your body to hold steady in this challenging pose whether agreeable or disagreeable; win mind control and find a measure of contentment in whatever comes your way.

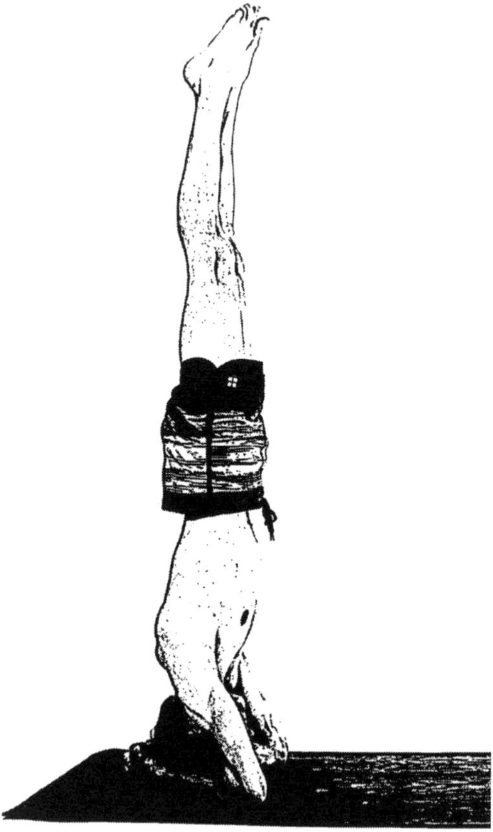

Śīrṣāsana
(Head Balance Pose)

— Line up your ankles, knees, hips and shoulders along an imaginary plumb line.

— Ground your forearms, wrists and hands; lift your shoulders and brace your upper back.

— Suck your lower front ribs into your body and widen your back ribs.

— Lengthen your tailbone; suck your navel back towards your spine and hollow your abdomen.

— Press your femur bones back and draw your sacrum forward.

— Activate these "Big 4" muscle groups in unison:
  1) Contract the fronts and backs of your thighs
  2) Firm your buttocks and engage your abdomen.

— Reach up through your legs with the power of a rocket launching into space.

— Direct the thrust of your legs vertically up through the bones from hips to toes.

— Constrict your throat and make a long steady sound as you empty your lungs; send life force up the axis to the base of your pelvis.

— Make a long steady sound as you fill up your lungs to the top of your chest; send vital energy down the axis to awaken your palate.

— Breathe skillfully along the axis to gain skill in recreating Samasthitiḥ in any pose.

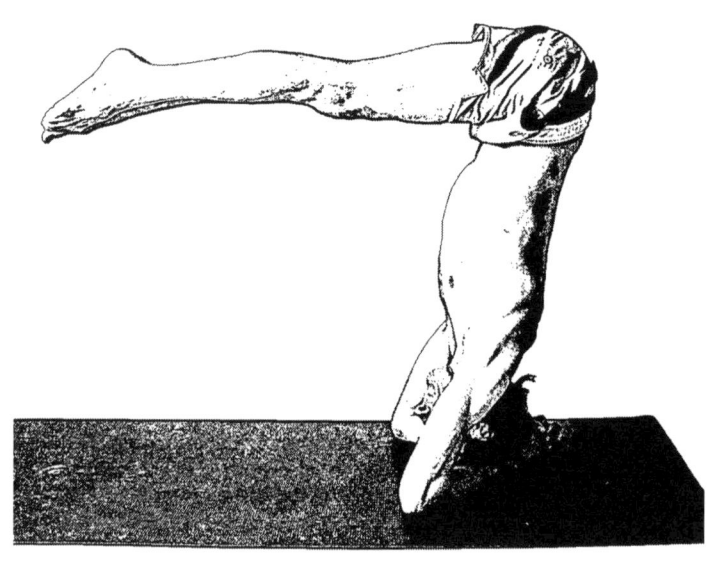

Ardha Śīrṣāsana
(Upward Staff Pose)

— Stamp the earth with your forearms, lift your shoulders, and brace your upper back.
— Kick forward horizontally with a mighty thrust through your leg bones.
— Elongate your legs with fiery intensity and open the backs of the knees to the sky.
— Contract your thigh muscles strongly and hug the muscles to the bones; make your legs powerful, dense, compact, solid, and yet alive with purpose and creativity.
— Gaze at a point on the ground or towards the horizon.
— Create an adamant upside down half pike position and strike the immovable spot.

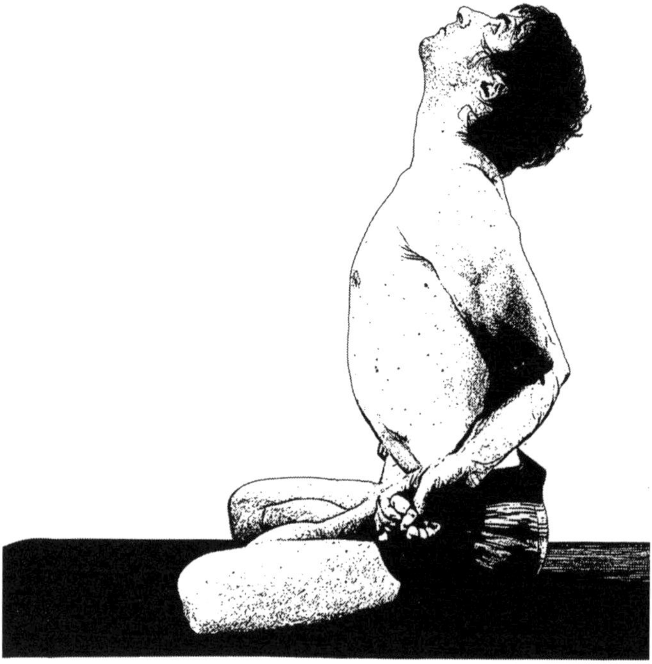

Baddha Padmāsana
(Bound Lotus Pose)

— Grip your feet with your hands and draw your elbows closer together.

— Suck your knees toward each other and stamp your legs down.

— Anchor your legs and vertically line up your head, torso, and pelvis.

— Pull up your navel and raise up Śakti from the base of your spine.

— Lift the pit of your abdomen and float the core of your heart.

— Roll back your shoulders and create a mighty expansion across your chest; throw your head back and kiss the sky.

— Alternately, bow your head and create a chin lock; send energy down the axis.

— Constrict your throat, and breathe with sound.

— Cast your gaze down into your heart center and find a lamp shining there lit by the flame of the Self, unwavering, smokeless, and never burning down.

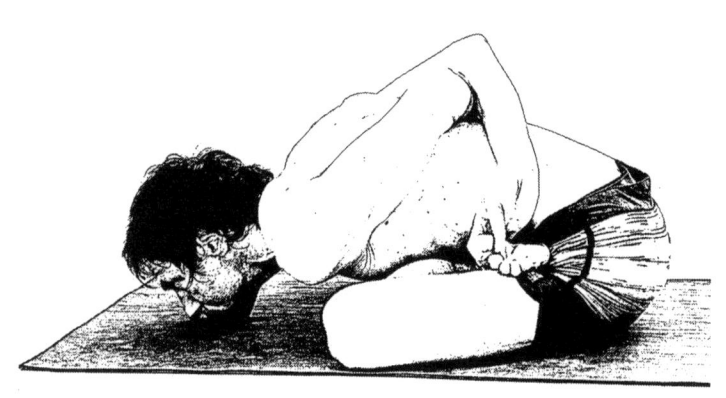

Yoga Mudrā
(Union Seal Pose)

— Increase the weight of your legs and pelvis; allow your anchored lower body to tether you to the earth.

— Grip your feet with your hands; project your torso forward and patiently elongate your spine from root to crown.

— Lower your forehead or chin to the ground and bow down to the beloved earth.

— Broaden your palate and cast an empty gaze between your eyebrows.

— Enjoy your legs bound in Lotus, your arms bound around your torso, and your feet bound by the grip of your hands.

— Seal in your life force and awaken the flow of creative energy inside your body.

— Remove gross movement; allow your limbs and three main body masses to stop and rest; then stop subtle movement; withdraw your senses to the deep interior and find absorption.

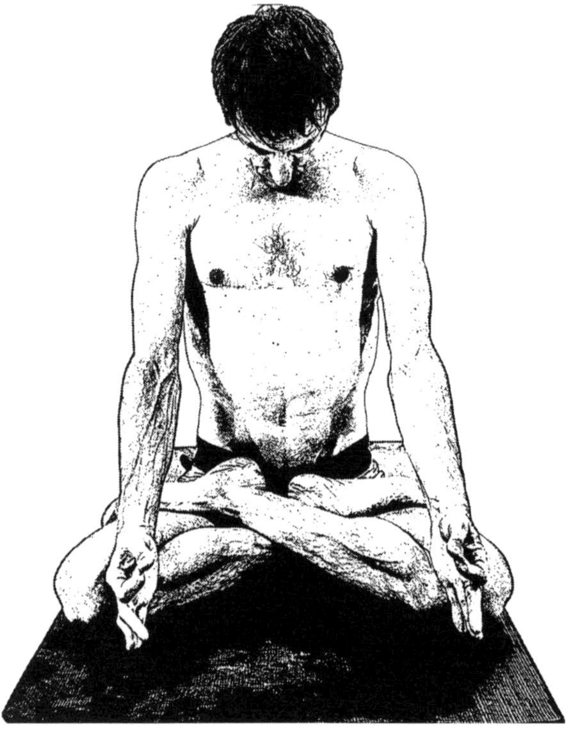

Ujjāyī in Padmāsana
(Victorious Breath in Lotus Pose)

— Breathe with sound and perform the three famous mudrās along the axis: Mūla, Uḍḍīyāna, and Jālandhara Bandhas.

— Constrict your throat; create resistance to the inflow and outflow of air; lengthen the breath by lengthening the sound; fill up and empty your lungs more thoroughly.

— Follow your breath's movements inside your body with great curiosity.

— Get creative; play with the length, speed, volume, rhythm, and pauses of each new cycle of breath.

— Direct the sound up and down the central axis between your pelvic floor and your palate.

— Send your mind down to the base of the axis within your pelvis as you finish emptying your lungs.

— Finish exhaling and create a gap before inhaling. During the pause fly your belly up into a hollow.

— Focus your mind at the sacred esoteric location known as the root of your palate, this will help you fill up your lungs with proper skill and tact.

— Pause after you finish inhaling. During the pause, lock your chin onto your chest and confine the expansion force of the inhalation within your body.

— Breathe and expertly sweep Prāṇa up and down the middle axis; succeed in moving Śakti and awaken the inherent wisdom faculty within you.

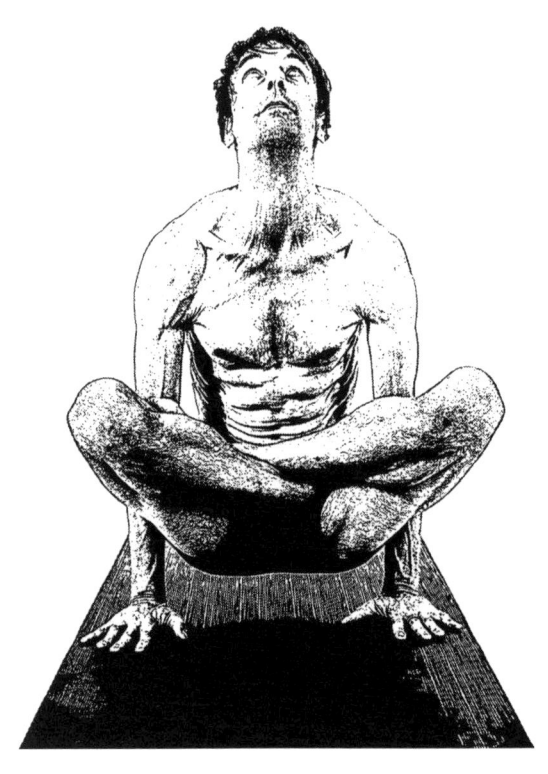

Utplutiḥ
(Sprung Up Pose)

— Plant your hands and lift up away from the earth.
— Strike down firmly through your hands; press your fingers and knuckles and ground your palms.
— Focus on lifting up your legs, then focus on lifting your seat, then lift both.
— Galvanize your core; pull up from the root of your spine and lift your navel.
— Lift up your legs and pelvis even if they are heavy or don't physically come up off the ground.
— Any effort brings great merit.
— Do the simple purification; stay up, hold your position, and build arm, core, and mental strength; breathe, and look up with a gaze of pure fire.

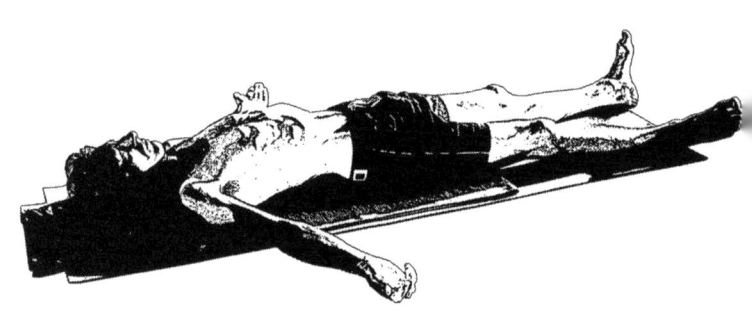

Śavāsana
(Corpse Pose)

— Lie back and relax; release all tension; allow your body to be fully supported by the earth.

— Let body and mind wind down to the earth and into stillness.

— Release your legs and arms; let your head and spine go; soften the heart center and release the belly.

— Withdraw your eyes and ears from outside to inside your body; gaze and listen within.

— Rest your senses; simply receive sense impressions without push or pull, action or reaction.

— The refuge you seek is inside of you; rest well and be at one within your very own body.

— Imagine that nothing but space exists within you; no muscles or bones, no desires or I-ness; only pure, unlimited space.

— Contemplate the word Śava, Corpse; cause all activity within your body and mind to disappear like a magician's trick; wink and become dead while living.

Copyright

Please email asanakitchen@gmail.com if you'd like to use any of this material in a training.

All rights reserved.

No part of this publication may be reproduced, stored in a retrieval system, stored in a database and/or published in any form or by any means, electronic, mechanical, photocopying, recording or otherwise, without the prior written permission of the publisher.

Made in the USA
Middletown, DE
08 June 2023